# Lung Disease in Rheumatic Diseases

*Editors*

ARYEH FISCHER
PAUL F. DELLARIPA

# RHEUMATIC DISEASE CLINICS OF NORTH AMERICA

www.rheumatic.theclinics.com

*Consulting Editor*
MICHAEL H. WEISMAN

May 2015 • Volume 41 • Number 2

**ELSEVIER**

1600 John F. Kennedy Boulevard ● Suite 1800 ● Philadelphia, Pennsylvania, 19103-2899
http://www.theclinics.com

RHEUMATIC DISEASE CLINICS OF NORTH AMERICA Volume 41, Number 2
May 2015 ISSN 0889-857X, ISBN 13: 978-0-323-37619-8

Editor: Jennifer Flynn-Briggs
Developmental Editor: Casey Jackson

*Rheumatic Disease Clinics of North America* (ISSN 0889-857X) is published quarterly by Elsevier Inc., 360 Park Avenue South, New York, NY 10010-1710. Months of issue are February, May, August, and November. Business and editorial offices: 1600 John F. Kennedy Boulevard, Suite 1800, Philadelphia, PA 19103-2899. Periodicals postage paid at New York, NY and additional mailing offices. Subscription prices are USD 335.00 per year for US individuals, USD 579.00 per year for US institutions, USD 165.00 per year for US students and residents, USD 395.00 per year for Canadian individuals, USD 722.00 per year for Canadian institutions, USD 465.00 per year for international individuals, USD 722.00 per year for international institutions, and USD 230.00 per year for Canadian and foreign students/residents. To receive student/resident rate, orders must be accompanied by name of affiliated institution, date of term, and the *signature* of program/residency coordinator on institution letterhead. Orders will be billed at individual rate until proof of status received. Foreign air speed delivery is included in all *Clinics* subscription prices. All prices are subject to change without notice. **POSTMASTER:** Send address changes to *Rheumatic Disease Clinics of North America,* Elsevier Health Sciences Division, Subscription Customer Service, 3251 Riverport Lane, Maryland Heights, MO 63043. **Customer Service: 1-800-654-2452 (US and Canada). From outside of the US and Canada: 314-447-8871. Fax: 314-447-8029. For print support, e-mail: JournalsCustomerService-usa@elsevier.com**. **For online support, e-mail: JournalsOnline Support-usa@elsevier.com**.

*Reprints.* For copies of 100 or more of articles in this publication, please contact the Commercial Reprints Department, Elsevier Inc., 360 Park Avenue South, New York, New York, 10010-1710; Tel.: +1-212-633-3874, Fax: +1-212-633-3820, and E-mail: reprints@elsevier.com.

*Rheumatic Disease Clinics of North America* is covered in *MEDLINE/PubMed (Index Medicus), Current Contents/Clinical Medicine, Science Citation Index, ISI/BIOMED,* and *EMBASE/Excerpta Medica.*

# Contributors

## CONSULTING EDITOR

**MICHAEL H. WEISMAN, MD**
Cedars-Sinai Chair in Rheumatology, Director, Division of Rheumatology, Professor of Medicine, Cedars-Sinai Medical Center, Distinguished Professor of Medicine, David Geffen School of Medicine at UCLA, Los Angeles, California

## EDITORS

**ARYEH FISCHER, MD**
Associate Professor of Medicine, Department of Medicine, National Jewish Health, University of Colorado School of Medicine, Denver, Colorado

**PAUL F. DELLARIPA, MD**
Division of Rheumatology, Brigham and Women's Hospital, Associate Professor of Medicine, Harvard Medical School, Boston, Massachusetts

## AUTHORS

**ANDY ABRIL, MD**
Assistant Professor, Department of Rheumatology, Mayo Clinic, Jacksonville, Florida

**DANA P. ASCHERMAN, MD**
Associate Professor of Medicine, Division of Rheumatology, University of Miami Miller School of Medicine, Miami, Florida

**DEBORAH ASSAYAG, MDCM, FRCPC**
Department of Medicine, McGill University, Montreal, Quebec, Canada

**FLAVIA V. CASTELINO, MD**
Division of Rheumatology, Massachusetts General Hospital; Assistant Professor of Medicine, Harvard Medical School, Boston, Massachusetts

**SANDRA CHARTRAND, MD, FRCPC**
Department of Medicine, National Jewish Health, Rheumatology Research Fellow, University of Colorado School of Medicine, Denver, Colorado; Department of Medicine, Rheumatology Clinic, Hôpital Maisonneuve-Rosemont, Université de Montréal, Montréal, Quebec, Canada

**LORINDA CHUNG, MD, MS**
Associate Professor, Division of Rheumatology and Immunology, Stanford University School of Medicine, Stanford, California; VA Palo Alto Health Care System, Palo Alto, California

**SUJAL R. DESAI, MD, FRCP, FRCR**
Consultant Radiologist and Honorary Senior Lecturer, Department of Radiology, King's College Hospital, London, United Kingdom

**ARYEH FISCHER, MD**
Associate Professor of Medicine, Department of Medicine, National Jewish Health, University of Colorado School of Medicine, Denver, Colorado

**MARILYN K. GLASSBERG, MD**
Professor of Medicine, Division of Pulmonary, Allergy, Critical Care, and Sleep Medicine, University of Miami Miller School of Medicine, Miami, Florida

**LINDSAY LALLY, MD**
Assistant Professor of Medicine, Division of Rheumatology, Hospital for Special Surgery, New York, New York

**SHELLY A. MILLER, MD**
Fellow, Division of Pulmonary, Allergy, Critical Care, and Sleep Medicine, University of Miami Miller School of Medicine, Miami, Florida

**ISABEL C. MIRA-AVENDANO, MD**
Assistant Professor, Department of Pulmonary Medicine, Mayo Clinic, Jacksonville, Florida

**ARJUN NAIR, MD, MRCP, FRCR**
Consultant Radiologist, Department of Radiology, Guy's and St Thomas' NHS Foundation Trust, London, United Kingdom

**ROBERT F. PADERA, MD, PhD**
Department of Pathology, Brigham and Women's Hospital, Boston, Massachusetts

**CHRISTOPHER J. RYERSON, MD, FRCPC**
Department of Medicine, St. Paul's Hospital, University of British Columbia, Vancouver, British Columbia, Canada

**SARA R. SCHOENFELD, MD**
Fellow, Division of Rheumatology, Massachusetts General Hospital, Boston, Massachusetts

**JOSHUA J. SOLOMON, MD**
Assistant Professor, Department of Medicine, Autoimmune Lung Center, National Jewish Health, Denver, Colorado

**ROBERT F. SPIERA, MD**
Professor of Medicine, Division of Rheumatology, Hospital for Special Surgery, New York, New York

**YON K. SUNG, MD**
Clinical Instructor, Division of Pulmonary and Critical Care Medicine, Vera Moulton Wall Center for Pulmonary Vascular Disease, Stanford University School of Medicine, Stanford, California

**MARINA VIVERO, MD**
Department of Pathology, Brigham and Women's Hospital, Boston, Massachusetts

**SIMON L.F. WALSH, MD, MRCP, FFRRCSI**
Consultant Cardiothoracic Radiologist, King's College Hospital, London, United Kingdom

**ZULMA X. YUNT, MD**
Assistant Professor, Department of Medicine, Autoimmune Lung Center, National Jewish Health, Denver, Colorado

# Contents

Lung disease commonly occurs in connective tissue diseases (CTD) and is an important cause of morbidity and mortality. Imaging is central to the evaluation of CTD-associated pulmonary complications. In this article, a general discussion of radiologic considerations is followed by a description of the pulmonary appearances in individual CTDs, and the imaging appearances of acute and nonacute pulmonary complications. The contribution of imaging to monitoring disease, evaluating treatment response, and prognostication is reviewed. Finally, we address the role of imaging in the challenging multidisciplinary evaluation of interstitial lung disease where there is an underlying suspicion of an undiagnosed CTD.

The pathologic correlates of interstitial lung disease (ILD) secondary to connective tissue disease (CTD) comprise a diverse group of histologic patterns. Lung biopsies in patients with CTD-associated ILD tend to demonstrate simultaneous involvement of multiple anatomic compartments of the lung. Certain histologic patterns tend to predominate in each defined CTD, and it is possible in many cases to confirm connective tissue-associated lung disease and guide patient management using surgical lung biopsy. This article will cover the pulmonary pathologies seen in rheumatoid arthritis, systemic sclerosis, myositis, systemic lupus erythematosus, Sjögren syndrome, and mixed CTD.

Connective tissue diseases (CTDs) can affect the lungs through diseases of the chest wall, pleura, vasculature, airways, and parenchyma. Interstitial lung disease (ILD) is a common complication of CTD associated with increased morbidity and mortality. This article describes the evaluation of respiratory impairment in patients with CTD and summarizes the evidence that guides diagnosis and management of CTD-ILD. Patients with CTD with suspected ILD should undergo clinical, physiologic, and radiologic studies to evaluate for the presence of ILD, and these results should be integrated in a multidisciplinary setting to guide diagnosis and management. Screening for ILD may also be appropriate in asymptomatic patients with high-risk features.

Rheumatoid arthritis (RA) affects approximately 1% of the US population frequently has extra-articular manifestations. Most compartments of the lung are susceptible to disease. Interstitial lung disease (ILD) and airways disease are the most common forms of RA-related lung disease. RA-ILD carries the worst prognosis and most often manifests in a histologic pattern of usual interstitial pneumonia or nonspecific interstitial pneumonia. There have been no large, well-controlled prospective studies investigating therapies for RA-ILD. Treatment usually entails immunomodulatory agents. Further studies are needed to better understand pathogenic mechanisms of disease that lead to lung involvement in these patients.

Systemic sclerosis is a heterogeneous disease of unknown etiology with limited effective therapies. It is characterized by autoimmunity, vasculopathy, and fibrosis and is clinically manifested by multiorgan involvement. Interstitial lung disease is a common complication of systemic sclerosis and is associated with significant morbidity and mortality. The diagnosis of interstitial lung disease hinges on careful clinical evaluation and pulmonary function tests and high-resolution computed tomography. Effective therapeutic options are still limited. Several experimental therapies are currently in early-phase clinical trials and show promise.

Pulmonary complications cause significant morbidity and mortality in the idiopathic inflammatory myopathies. Advances in biomarker discovery have facilitated clinical phenotyping, allowing investigators to better define at-risk patient subsets and to potentially gauge disease activity. This serologic characterization has complemented more traditional assessment tools. Pharmacologic management continues to rely on the use of corticosteroids, often in combination with additional immunosuppressive agents. The rarity of myositis-associated interstitial lung disease and lack of controlled trials have limited analyses of treatment efficacy, mandating the development of standardized outcome measures and improvement of data sharing between disciplines.

Interstitial lung disease is a common and often life-threatening manifestation of different connective tissue disorders, often affecting its overall prognosis. Systemic lupus erythematosus, Sjögren syndrome, and mixed connective tissue disease, although all unique diseases, can have lung manifestations as an important part of these conditions. This article reviews the different pulmonary manifestations seen in these 3 systemic rheumatologic conditions.

A thorough, often multidisciplinary assessment to determine extrathoracic versus intrathoracic disease activity and degrees of impairment is needed to optimize the management of connective tissue disease (CTD)–associated interstitial lung disease (ILD). Pharmacologic intervention with immunosuppression is the mainstay of therapy for all forms of CTD-ILD, but should be reserved for those that show clinically significant and/or progressive disease. The management of CTD-ILD is not yet evidence based and there is a need for controlled trials across the spectrum of CTD-ILD. Nonpharmacologic management strategies and addressing comorbidities or aggravating factors should be included in the comprehensive treatment plan for CTD-ILD.

Pulmonary arterial hypertension (PAH) is characterized by vascular remodeling of pulmonary arterioles that leads to increased pulmonary vascular resistance, right heart failure, and death. It is associated with connective tissue diseases, including systemic sclerosis, systemic lupus erythematosus, and mixed connective tissue disease. PAH is characterized by dyspnea on exertion and fatigue. Syncopal events suggest severe disease. Patients may present with signs of right heart failure. One- and 3-year survival rates are approximately 81% and 52%, respectively. Given the high prevalence and mortality, algorithms for screening are currently under investigation and will hopefully lead to earlier diagnosis and improved survival.

Pulmonary vasculitis encompasses inflammation in the pulmonary vasculature with involved vessels varying in caliber from large elastic arteries to capillaries. Small pulmonary capillaries are the vessels most commonly involved in vasculitis affecting the lung. The antineutrophil cytoplasmic antibody–associated vasculitides, which include granulomatosis with polyangiitis (formerly Wegener granulomatosis), microscopic polyangiitis, and eosinophilic granulomatosis with polyangiitis (formerly Churg-Strauss syndrome), are the small vessel vasculitides in which pulmonary vasculitis is most frequently observed and are the major focus of this review. Vasculitic involvement of the large pulmonary vessels as may occur in Behçet syndrome and Takayasu arteritis is also discussed.

# RHEUMATIC DISEASE CLINICS
# OF NORTH AMERICA

---

**RELATED INTEREST**

*Cardiology Clinics,* February 2015 (Volume 33, Issue 1)
**Preoperative Cardiovascular Evaluation in Patients Undergoing Vascular Surgery**
Parveen K. Garg, *Editor*

---

DOWNLOAD
Free App!

*Review Articles*
THE CLINICS

**NOW AVAILABLE FOR YOUR iPhone and iPad**

# Foreword

# Lung Disease in Rheumatic Diseases

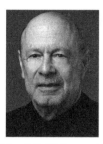

Michael H. Weisman, MD
*Consulting Editor*

Aryeh and Paul have created a unique volume that should be a reference standard for years to come regarding disease description, pathogenesis, and treatment of the pulmonary associations and complications of our rheumatic disease patients. The literature is reviewed carefully and the recommendations from the various article writers are clear, well thought-out, and evidence-based. For many years, the lung-associated conditions related to our diseases were relegated to the backwaters of investigation, surviving in the literature as only descriptions of late-stage complications or even curiosities without pathologic significance. Now that many of our diseases (rheumatoid arthritis, in particular) are diagnosed at an early stage and clearly treated more effectively, the paradoxical effect is that pulmonary complications have become more prominent clinically, especially regarding outcome. Increased safety for obtaining lung tissue for direct examination as well as advanced imaging techniques made available everywhere has enabled many of these advances. In addition, since the lung is one of the major portals of entry for potential environmental triggers of rheumatic diseases, recent investigations are now focusing on the lung for early mucosal dysregulation effects that perpetuate the chronicity of our diseases. This volume covers much of these issues for the clinician, investigator, student, resident, and fellow. Read all about it.

Michael H. Weisman, MD
Division of Rheumatology
Cedars-Sinai Medical Center
8700 Beverly Boulevard
Los Angeles, CA 90024, USA

E-mail address:
Michael.Weisman@cshs.org

Rheum Dis Clin N Am 41 (2015) xi
http://dx.doi.org/10.1016/j.rdc.2015.03.002
0889-857X/15/$ – see front matter © 2015 Published by Elsevier Inc.

**rheumatic.theclinics.com**

# Preface

# Demystifying Lung Disease in the Rheumatic Diseases

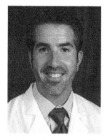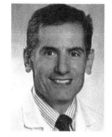

Aryeh Fischer, MD        Paul F. Dellaripa, MD
*Editors*

This issue of *Rheumatic Disease Clinics of North America* is dedicated to Lung Disease in Rheumatic Diseases and aims to provide a practical resource, with a multidisciplinary emphasis, for the practicing clinician to optimize the evaluation and management of lung disease in rheumatic diseases.

There is a myriad of pulmonary manifestations, with varied incidence and prevalence, associated with the rheumatic diseases; essentially every component of the respiratory tract is at risk of injury in these patients. Furthermore, despite the remarkable advances over the past decades in managing rheumatic diseases, lung disease continues to be associated with significant morbidity and is a leading cause of mortality in patients with rheumatic disease. It is not known why some rheumatic diseases are more likely to be associated with certain types of lung involvement, and there is much to learn about the natural history and treatment of lung involvement among these cohorts.

For the clinician, the evaluation of the rheumatic disease patient with cough or dyspnea and diffusely abnormal chest imaging is always a challenge. The clinical context, pulmonary physiology data, the patterns visualized on thoracic high-resolution computerized tomographic scanning, and the histopathologic findings on lung biopsy specimens all play a critical role in the search for the diagnosis. We start with a practical and thorough overview of the radiologist's approach to lung disease in rheumatic disease patients followed by a comprehensive review of the pulmonary histopathologic patterns identified in these cohorts. Moving beyond imaging and pathology, with hopes of providing a map for this clinical maze and highlighting the importance of each piece of information and where it fits—the approach to determining respiratory impairment in those with rheumatic diseases is provided. The subsequent articles review the specific rheumatic diseases and their associated forms of lung

Rheum Dis Clin N Am 41 (2015) xiii–xiv
http://dx.doi.org/10.1016/j.rdc.2015.03.001
0889-857X/15/$ – see front matter © 2015 Published by Elsevier Inc.

**rheumatic.theclinics.com**

disease. Specifically, the lung manifestations of rheumatoid arthritis, systemic sclerosis, poly-/dermatomyositis, systemic lupus erythematosus, mixed connective tissue disease, and Sjögren syndrome are comprehensively discussed. A practical approach to the comprehensive management of interstitial lung disease in patients with rheumatic diseases is then provided. The final two articles provide an up-to-date and thorough review of pulmonary hypertension associated with rheumatic diseases and pulmonary vasculitis.

We recognize the outstanding combined efforts of the authors of this thematic issue for *Rheumatic Disease Clinics of North America* and hope this volume serves to further your understanding of the complex intersection of lung disease in rheumatic diseases and proves to be a useful resource that enhances your care of these patients.

Aryeh Fischer, MD
National Jewish Health
University of Colorado School of Medicine
1400 Jackson Street, G07
Denver, CO 80206, USA

Paul F. Dellaripa, MD
Division of Rheumatology
Brigham and Women's Hospital
Harvard Medical School
75 Francis Street
Boston, MA 02115, USA

E-mail addresses:
fischera@njhealth.org (A. Fischer)
pdellaripa@partners.org (P.F. Dellaripa)

# Imaging of Pulmonary Involvement in Rheumatic Disease

Arjun Nair, MD, MRCP, FRCR[a], Simon L.F. Walsh, MD, MRCP, FFRRCSI[b],
Sujal R. Desai, MD, FRCP, FRCR[c],*

## KEYWORDS

- Computed tomography • Imaging • Connective tissue diseases
- Interstitial lung diseases

## KEY POINTS

- There is a high degree of overlap between the pulmonary manifestations of the various connective tissue diseases (CTDs), particularly with respect to interstitial lung disease (ILD) patterns.
- Nonspecific interstitial pneumonia (NSIP) is the most common ILD pattern in all CTDs apart from rheumatoid arthritis, where usual interstitial pneumonia (UIP) is the most frequent pattern.
- Distinguishing between acute exacerbation, infection, drug toxicity, or pulmonary hemorrhage as the cause for acute deterioration in CTD-associated lung disease is impossible on high-resolution computed tomography (HRCT) appearances alone, but requires the integration of clinical and serologic data with the evolution of appearances on plain radiograph.
- A role for HRCT in staging disease and aiding prognostication has recently been shown, with traction bronchiectasis and extent of honeycombing both associated with increased mortality in CTD-ILD.

## INTRODUCTION

The rheumatic diseases are a heterogeneous group of inflammatory disorders characterized principally by joint disease, but also, not infrequently, multiorgan dysfunction. Lung disease is common in connective tissue diseases (CTDs) and is an important

Disclosure Statement: All authors have nothing to disclose.
[a] Department of Radiology, Guy's and St Thomas' NHS Foundation Trust, Great Maze Pond, London SE1 9RT, UK; [b] Department of Radiology, King's College Hospital, Denmark Hill, London SE5 9RS, UK; [c] Department of Radiology, King's College Hospital, Denmark Hill, London SE5 9RS, UK
* Corresponding author. Department of Radiology, King's College Hospital, Denmark Hill, London SE5 9RS, UK.
E-mail address: sujal.desai@nhs.net

Rheum Dis Clin N Am 41 (2015) 167–196
http://dx.doi.org/10.1016/j.rdc.2014.12.001
0889-857X/15/$ – see front matter © 2015 Elsevier Inc. All rights reserved.

rheumatic.theclinics.com

cause of both morbidity and mortality. The CTDs (sometimes termed collagen vascular diseases) include rheumatoid arthritis (RA), systemic sclerosis (SSc), systemic lupus erythematosus (SLE), polymyositis/dermatomyositis (PM/DM), primary Sjögren syndrome (SS), mixed connective tissue disease (MCTD), and undifferentiated connective tissue disease (UCTD). Radiologic assessment has a definite role in the management of CTD-associated pulmonary disease. In this regard, plain chest radiography and high-resolution computed tomography (HRCT) are the principal tests. The indications for imaging will vary, but a typical scenario for the radiologist is to establish whether lung disease is present and, if so, to characterize its nature and extent. In cases in which a histospecific radiologic diagnosis of lung disease cannot be provided, HRCT may be the best guide to the optimal site for surgical biopsy. More recently, there has been interest in the utility of HRCT to assess longitudinal behavior and prognosis.

In the present article, a general discussion of radiologic features is followed by a description of the appearances in individual CTDs. We then consider the pulmonary complications of CTDs on imaging, the use of imaging in prognostication, and the role of multidisciplinary evaluation. Given the acknowledged limitations of plain chest radiography in characterizing patterns of diffuse lung disease in general[1,2] and in CTD-associated lung disorders,[3–5] the article focuses primarily on HRCT appearances. Pulmonary involvement also occurs in other rheumatic disorders, such as vasculitides and inflammatory disorders, including spondyloarthropathy, Behçet disease, and relapsing polychondritis, but the thoracic radiologic manifestations of these conditions are distinct from the CTDs listed previously and are outside the scope of this article.

## GENERAL RADIOLOGIC AND PATHOLOGIC CONSIDERATIONS

The CTDs can affect the pulmonary and extrapulmonary components of the thorax to varying degrees. The main manifestations in the pulmonary interstitium, airspaces, airways, pulmonary vasculature, pleura, pericardium, heart, mediastinum, and thoracic musculature are given in **Table 1**. Among the thoracic manifestations of the CTDs, the interstitial diseases are perhaps the most intriguing and widely studied. In this regard, an important consideration is that almost all the patterns of idiopathic interstitial pneumonias (IIPs) (but, importantly, not their prevalences), are mirrored in CTD-related interstitial lung disease (ILD). The radiologic and histopathologic features of the IIPs have been well documented (**Table 2**).[6–8] Indeed, it may be argued that the true utility

**Table 1**
**Thoracic manifestations of the connective tissue disorders**

| Compartment | Manifestation |
|---|---|
| Airways | Bronchial wall thickening, bronchiectasis, obliterative bronchiolitis |
| Lung parenchyma | Interstitial lung disease: interstitial pneumonias (see **Table 2**)<br>Airspace disease: diffuse alveolar damage, pulmonary hemorrhage<br>Necrobiotic nodules, infection, malignancy |
| Pulmonary vasculature | Acute/chronic pulmonary thromboembolism, pulmonary hypertension |
| Pleura/pericardium | Pleural/pericardial thickening, nodularity or effusion, pneumothorax |
| Mediastinum | Esophageal dilatation/dysfunction, enlarged mediastinal lymph nodes |
| Thoracic musculature | Muscle dysfunction leading to ventilatory impairment |

**Table 2**
High-resolution computed tomography (HRCT) and histopathological characteristics of the interstitial pneumonias encountered in connective tissue diseases

| Pattern | HRCT Features | Histopathologic Features | Remarks |
|---|---|---|---|
| Usual interstitial pneumonia (UIP) | • Subpleural basal predominant reticulation<br>• Honeycombing ± traction bronchiectasis<br>• GGO usually inconspicuous | • Marked fibrosis, architectural distortion<br>• ± Subpleural/paraseptal predominant honeycombing<br>• Patchy involvement<br>• Fibroblastic foci<br>• Only mild interstitial inflammatory infiltrate | Criteria for definite, possible, and inconsistent with UIP (on both HRCT and pathology) and probable UIP (on pathology only) have been defined |
| Nonspecific interstitial pneumonia (NSIP) | • Bilateral GGO<br>• Some basal and subpleural predominance<br>• Fine reticulation/irregular linear opacities<br>• ± Traction bronchiectasis/bronchiolectasis<br>• Honeycombing sparse/absent | • Varying amounts of interstitial inflammation and fibrosis<br>• Uniform appearance | Honeycombing may become more prominent with progression<br>Katzenstein grades of pure cellular (grade I), mixed cellular and fibrotic (grade II), and fibrotic (grade III) recognized histopathologically |
| Organizing pneumonia (OP) | • Patchy, multifocal consolidation<br>• Subpleural or peribronchial distribution<br>• May be associated with GGO, perilobular pattern<br>• ± Centrilobular nodules or masses | • Intraluminal plugs of inflammatory debris: buds of granulation tissue and Masson bodies (whorls of fibroblasts and myofibroblasts in a connective matrix)<br>• Predominantly within the alveolar ducts and surrounding alveoli<br>• Mild interstitial inflammation | May coexist with an NSIP pattern |
| Lymphocytic interstitial pneumonia (LIP) | • Ill-defined GGO and centrilobular nodules<br>• Peribronchial/interlobular septal thickening<br>• Thin-walled perivascular cysts<br>• ± Lymph node enlargement | • Diffuse interstitial infiltration: mostly T-lymphocytes, plasma cells, and macrophages<br>• Predominantly alveolar septal distribution<br>• Frequent bronchial mucosa-associated lymphoid tissue hyperplasia | Can be regarded as interstitial-predominant variant of diffuse pulmonary lymphoid hyperplasia<br>Follicular bronchiolitis is another form of predominantly peribronchial/peribronchiolar lymphocytic infiltrate seen in rheumatoid arthritis |

*Abbreviation:* GGO, ground-glass opacity.
*Adapted from* Refs.[6–8]

of HRCT is not in predicting the underlying CTD (because this invariably requires the integration of clinical, serologic, and radiologic data), but in identifying the likely pattern of interstitial pneumonia, which not only has prognostic implications but also may influence the decision to biopsy. In this regard, it is important to stress that overlapping HRCT appearances (particularly for usual interstitial pneumonia [UIP] and nonspecific interstitial pneumonia [NSIP][9–11]) are not uncommon; predominant ground-glass opacification is the important feature of NSIP,[9,12] whereas the cardinal findings in UIP are subpleural, basal reticulation with honeycombing.[7,13,14] In the absence of honeycombing, attempting to make a radiologic diagnosis of "possible" UIP rather than NSIP relies on the observation of less extensive ground-glass attenuation compared with coarse reticulation with a subpleural, basal predominance, and the absence of the other features inconsistent with UIP.[7] However, the use of such an interpretation algorithm can still result in misdiagnosis of biopsy-proven NSIP as UIP on HRCT, and vice-versa.[11,15] It is also worth stating that inter-reader agreement for honeycombing is, at best, fair to moderate[16–18] and that differentiating honeycombing from peripheral traction bronchiolectasis, on transaxial interspaced HRCT images, is not straightforward.[16,19]

In addition to what has already been stated previously, some general comments about the imaging of CTD-related ILD also can be made. First, with the notable exception of RA (in which a UIP pattern is most prevalent[20,21]), NSIP is the dominant pattern of CTD-related ILD.[22,23] Second, the presence of either mixed HRCT patterns (eg, features of lung fibrosis together with consolidation) or the coexistence of an ILD with, say, signs of pleural or airways disease, should alert the radiologist to the possibility of an underlying CTD, particularly when extrapulmonary abnormalities are present.[24] Third, the notion that ground-glass opacification on HRCT denotes potentially reversible or treatable disease[25,26] is no longer considered true for the idiopathic interstitial pneumonias[27–29] or the CTD-related ILDs.[30,31] Ground-glass opacification may indicate fine fibrosis,[32] particularly when there is traction bronchiectasis/bronchiolectasis. The obvious message is that the mere presence of ground-glass attenuation should not be used as justification for potentially toxic therapy.

## IMAGING OF INDIVIDUAL CONNECTIVE TISSUE DISEASES
### Rheumatoid Arthritis

The pulmonary and pleural manifestations of RA have continued to receive attention ever since the early report from 1948 by Ellman and Ball.[33] The true prevalence of RA-associated thoracic disease is difficult to predict, chiefly because of differences in the populations studied and discordance between HRCT findings and symptoms. With respect to RA-related ILD, Gabbay and colleagues[3] reported that, in a population of 36 patients with joint manifestations of recent (2 years) onset, one-third had HRCT manifestations of ILD, but there was clinically significant disease in only 14%. However, when clinically significant ILD was defined as RA-associated ILD that contributes to death, Olson and colleagues[34] found that the prevalence of such ILD was closer to 7% in women and just less than 10% in men. The lifetime risk of developing ILD in patients with RA has been estimated at 7.7%.[35] In another study of patients with RA having one or more of symptomatic ILD, abnormal pulmonary function tests, or chest radiographs, Biederer and colleagues[36] found some form of HRCT abnormality in 92% of patients. As such, the prevalence of HRCT abnormalities is undeniably greater than the proportion with clinically relevant pulmonary disease.

### Airway disease

In patients with RA, airway abnormalities are common. Bronchiectasis, with or without bronchial wall thickening, may be seen in up to 30% of patients (**Fig. 1**).[36–41] Peripheral branching nodular opacities (the tree-in-bud pattern) and heterogeneity in lung density (the so-called mosaic attenuation pattern), both indicating involvement of small airways, also are relatively frequently seen on HRCT.[20,40,42–45] In one study of 50 patients with no evidence of RA-associated ILD, Perez and colleagues,[40] identified bronchiectasis in 30%, with a third of such cases associated with bronchial wall thickening. It is also noteworthy that, with time, the extent of bronchiectasis and severity of bronchial thickening generally worsens with long-standing RA.[46] The tree-in-bud pattern on HRCT indicates intraluminal/peribronchial small airway exudate and is reported in approximately 10% to 20% of patients with RA (**Fig. 2**).[20,43,44] Tree-in-bud opacities with centrilobular nodules also are seen in the rare entity of follicular bronchiolitis, which is characterized histologically by peribronchial lymphoid hyperplasia.[47–49] Indirect evidence of small airways disease, reflected on HRCT by mosaic attenuation, is present in 44% to 52% of cases (**Fig. 3**).[40,42] Although patients with this HRCT pattern may be asymptomatic, a subset with the functional entity of obliterative bronchiolitis in RA, as first reported by Geddes and colleagues,[50] experience rapidly progressive dyspnea and airflow obstruction.[42]

### Interstitial lung disease

It is now accepted that a pattern of UIP is more common than NSIP in patients with RA, despite earlier reports of equal[51] or higher[22] prevalence of NSIP. Although Tanaka and colleagues[20] reported that HRCT findings accurately reflect histopathologic features, in most cases the concordance between histopathologic and HRCT diagnosis can vary. Indeed, Lee and colleagues[52] demonstrated a histopathologic UIP pattern in

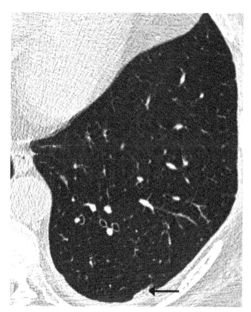

**Fig. 1.** A 69-year-old man with a long-standing history of RA. HRCT demonstrates minimal bronchial wall thickening and cylindrical bronchiectasis, together with some nonspecific pleural thickening (*arrow*).

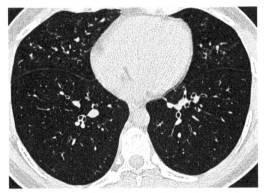

**Fig. 2.** A 41-year-old woman with a short history of RA and recent increasing cough. Transverse HRCT slice demonstrates quite marked centrilobular nodularity in the middle lobe and lingula, suspicious for an exudative small airways infection or follicular bronchiolitis. Mild cylindrical bronchiectasis and bronchial wall thickening are also noted.

10 (56%) of 18 patients with RA, 9 of whom demonstrated HRCT-concordant UIP with subpleural reticulation and honeycombing (**Fig. 4**A). By way of contrast, a more recent study,[52] which used the stricter HRCT definition of "definite UIP,"[7] resulted in only 19 (45%) of 42 histopathologically proven cases of UIP being radiologically classified as UIP.[53] Broadening the UIP definition to include cases of possible UIP (see **Fig. 4**B) improved the HRCT sensitivity for a UIP diagnosis to 81%, but at the expense of a diminished specificity and poorer agreement between radiologists. The variation in radiologic-pathologic concordance is undoubtedly due to differences in the proportions of patients with honeycombing, but this variation cannot easily be explained

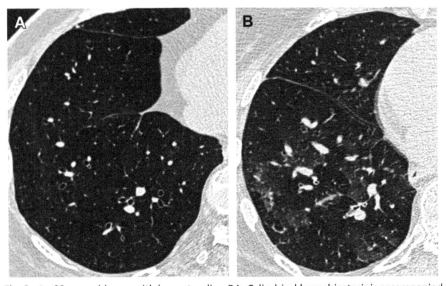

**Fig. 3.** An 88-year-old man with long-standing RA. Cylindrical bronchiectasis is accompanied by mild mosaic attenuation on inspiration (A), accentuated on expiratory imaging (B), due to air-trapping.

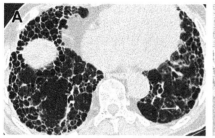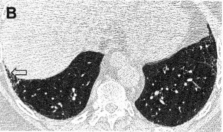

**Fig. 4.** HRCT for ILD in 2 patients with RA. (*A*) In a 73-year-old man with increasing breathlessness, a transverse HRCT slice demonstrates the definite UIP pattern of subpleural basal predominant honeycombing and traction bronchiectasis (*arrow*). (*B*) In a 74-year-old woman with recurrent cough, the HRCT demonstrates only minor subpleural reticulation and no definite traction bronchiectasis, but no features inconsistent with UIP. Honeycombing at the extreme base (*block arrow*) was thought to be present by one radiologist but not another at multidisciplinary discussion; a radiologic pattern of possible but not definite UIP was assigned.

by the duration of disease, as honeycombing may be present in equal proportions in both early and long-standing RA.[46]

There is an important possible link between smoking and pulmonary fibrosis in patients with RA. It would appear that tobacco smoke predisposes to RA-associated ILD,[54,55] particularly UIP over NSIP,[31,52] although the prognostic implications of smoking in RA-associated ILD are yet to be determined.[56,57] Intriguingly, a recent study demonstrated that emphysema, in both smokers with RA-associated ILD and smokers with idiopathic pulmonary fibrosis (IPF), was significantly more prevalent than in controls who smoked but who did not have chronic obstructive pulmonary disease (48% and 35% respectively, vs 15%), despite a lower pack-year smoking history.[58] This may be indirect evidence that shared mechanisms exist between smoking-related lung damage and RA-associated fibrosis.

In general, lung abnormalities in RA are either exclusively or predominantly present in the lower zones.[36,38,40,43,45] It is also worth noting that, that although ILD and airway abnormalities may coexist, one or the other usually predominates. In this regard, one hypothesis is that variability in human leukocyte antigen subtypes may predispose to bronchiectasis, rather than ILD, in RA.[39,41,59]

### Non–interstitial lung disease/airway manifestations of rheumatoid arthritis

Among the other recognized complications of RA in the chest, necrobiotic nodules (which have historically been considered a classic feature of RA-associated pulmonary involvement[60]) are surprisingly rare; the frequency and HRCT characteristics of necrobiotic nodules are difficult to ascertain because of a paucity of pathologic correlation. Pleural disease (usually pleural thickening rather than effusions), is common in RA, being present in up to 30% of patients on HRCT[36,38] and 50% in one autopsy series.[61] Enlarged mediastinal lymph nodes in RA also have been reported.[36]

### Systemic Sclerosis

#### Interstitial lung disease

ILD is prevalent in patients with SSc. Indeed, a higher prevalence of ILD on HRCT (reportedly between 36% and 91%[4,62–64]), is seen in SSc compared with the other CTDs. Pulmonary involvement contributes to mortality and ranks third in frequency behind cutaneous and peripheral vessel involvement in patients with SSc.[63] Although the extent of ILD on HRCT may vary between cases, limited disease is more common: in one large study of more than 200 patients, the median extent of abnormal lung was only 13% (range = 1%–84%),[65] reflecting, in part perhaps, the tendency for pulmonologists to "screen" patients for ILD.

It is now accepted that NSIP is more common than UIP as a pattern of ILD in SSc.[23,66] Other patterns of interstitial involvement, such as organizing pneumonia (OP),[67,68] are rare. In patients with SSc-associated NSIP, basal predominant subpleural ground-glass opacification with superimposed fine reticulation is the typical HRCT finding (**Figs. 5** and **6**).[30,69,70] Honeycombing may be present in up to 40% of cases[17,62,71] and, interestingly, appears to be more common in limited SSc.[17] Honeycombing tends to be limited in extent and characterized by a microcystic pattern. In one cohort of 52 patients with SSc with a median duration of 6.8 years of extrapulmonary disease, Remy-Jardin and colleagues[62] showed that 32 patients had abnormalities on HRCT: ground-glass opacification and a nonseptal linear pattern were present in 26 (50%) and 6 (12%) cases, respectively. When honeycombing was present, it was localized in most (12 of 19 cases, 63%). The extent of honeycombing can increase on serial HRCT and has been shown to correlate with a decline in the diffusion capacity for carbon monoxide (DLco).[62,72] From this, it is tempting to postulate that honeycombing is more prevalent in patients with disease of longer duration. However, no such relationship was observed in the study by Remy-Jardin and colleagues.[62] In addition, the observation on follow-up CT that ground-glass attenuation not only fails to resolve with treatment,[71,73] but is replaced by honeycombing,[62,71] supports the notion that ground-glass opacities may represent fine fibrosis rather than a predominantly cellular inflammatory infiltrate.[26]

A preponderance of ground-glass opacity, fibrosis of limited coarseness, and the relative absence of honeycombing should allow the differentiation of SSc-associated NSIP from patients with IPF. However, it must be remembered that the coarseness of fibrosis and extent of ground-glass opacity (relative to reticulation) may be similar in patients with idiopathic and SSc-associated NSIP, making discrimination between the latter 2 entities impossible on parenchymal appearances alone.[65] In practice, radiologists suspecting an HRCT pattern of NSIP may look for the other ancillary signs of diffuse SSc, such as esophageal dilatation or soft tissue calcinosis.

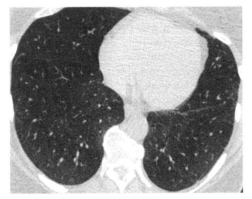

**Fig. 5.** A 55-year-old woman with a new diagnosis of SSc, exertional breathlessness, and DLco. Transverse HRCT slice demonstrates patchy, quite extensive pure ground-glass opacity with no admixed reticulation or traction bronchiectasis.

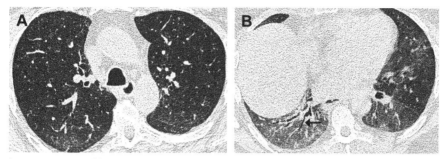

**Fig. 6.** A 62-year-old woman with known SSc and increasing breathlessness over 18 months. Transverse HRCT just below the aortic arch (*A*) and at the bases (*B*) demonstrate ground-glass opacity with some admixed reticulation in the upper lobes, becoming more predominant in the lower lobes where there has been quite marked volume loss (note the retracted position of the left oblique fissure) and traction bronchiectasis (*arrow* in *B*). Traction bronchiectasis is a poor prognostic sign.

### Non–interstitial lung disease manifestations of systemic sclerosis

Mediastinal lymph node enlargement, esophageal dilatation, and pleural abnormalities are the other CT abnormalities in patients with SSc. Nodal enlargement per se is seen in many diffuse lung diseases and has been correlated with the CT extent of ILD in SSc.[74–76] Esophageal dilatation is present in 62% to 82% of patients,[75,77,78] but whether or not esophageal dysmotility predisposes to, or correlates with, ILD is unclear.[79–81] Pleural abnormalities, manifest as subpleural micronodules or pleural thickening, are reported in as many as 81% of cases at autopsy,[82] but the frequency in HRCT studies is more variable.[62,72] Finally, for the sake of completeness, mention also is made of the complication of pulmonary hypertension in SSc, which is a key contributor to mortality, and is discussed in greater detail later in this article.

### Systemic lupus erythematosus

Lung disease in SLE is perhaps more prevalent than might first be appreciated; in one study, more than half of patients developed some feature of pleuroparenchymal involvement at some point during the course of disease.[83] Autopsy series suggest that pleural and pericardial abnormalities predominate[84,85]; however, the reported prevalence, based on radiologic investigations, has varied. For instance, Sant and colleagues[5] and Fenlon and colleagues[86] reported pericardial thickening and pleural involvement (ie, pleural tags, thickening, and effusions) in only 15% and 17% of HRCTs, respectively. By way of stark contrast, Ooi and colleagues[87] reported pleural disease in as many as 80%.

### Interstitial lung disease

Interstitial lung involvement (characterized by thickened interlobular septa, and parenchymal and subpleural bands) has been seen in 33% to 38% of patients with SLE, but, when present, is usually mild in extent and severity[86] and asymptomatic.[5] Against this, the preponderance of honeycombing and architectural distortion in just over half of patients with an HRCT-derived ILD diagnosis studied by Ooi and colleagues[87] is a salutary reminder of the influence of selection bias and small samples in many CTD-ILD studies. Indeed, it is believed that *symptomatic* ILD occurs in the minority (ie, <10%) of patients.[88,89] A possible caveat is that a higher prevalence of interstitial abnormalities has been noted in patients with the antiphospholipid syndrome, in which irregular subpleural linear opacities, ground-glass opacity, reticulation, and interlobular septal thickening are seen.[90] The more serious and potentially life-threatening complications of lupus pneumonitis and pulmonary hemorrhage are also recognized in SLE and are discussed in the section on pulmonary complications of CTD-associated disease.

An intriguing entity seen in patients with SLE that bears mentioning is "shrinking lung syndrome," characterized by unexplained and often progressive dyspnea, physiologic small-volume lungs, and diaphragmatic elevation but with clear lungs on plain radiograph (**Fig. 7**).[89–91] This clinico-radiologic constellation has been observed in approximately 10% of patients with SLE.[91–93] On HRCT there is bibasal atelectasis coupled with an elevated diaphragm. The pathogenesis of shrinking lungs remains unclear, but the role of primary diaphragmatic and/or respiratory muscle weakness (caused by a postulated subclinical myopathy[94,95]) is not supported by electrophysiologic data.[96,97]

### Polymyositis/dermatomyositis

In patients with PM/DM, lung disease can be problematic, and this is particularly true in the context of serum antibodies to aminoacyl-tRNA-synthetases (the so-called

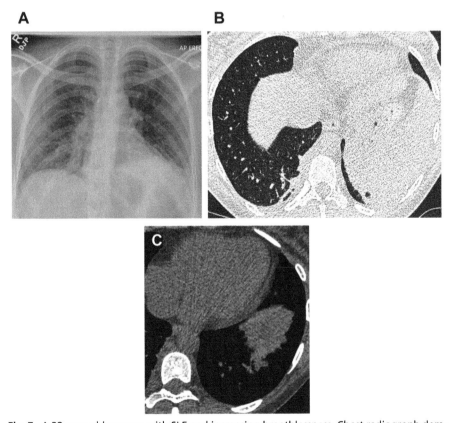

**Fig. 7.** A 38-year-old woman with SLE and increasing breathlessness. Chest radiograph demonstrates a raised left hemidiaphragm (*A*), whereas transverse HRCT on lung windows at the lung bases demonstrates the associated atelectasis at both bases in addition to the raised left hemidiaphragm (*B*), with some pericardial thickening as a sequelae of previous pericarditis also noted on mediastinal windows (*C*). The appearances were suspicious for the "shrinking lung" syndrome.

"antisynthetase" antibodies).[98,99] Of the antisynthetase syndromes, antibodies to histidyl-transfer RNA (more conveniently called anti-Jo1) are the most prevalent, and their importance is that ILD reportedly occurs in more than 50% of patients with anti-Jo1 positivity.[100–102]

The typical patterns of lung disease in PM/DM are NSIP and OP. Understandably, in most patients with ILD associated with PM/DM, the imaging features will reflect these patterns. Ground-glass opacification (present in 63%–92%) and consolidation (seen in 26%–55%) are frequently present, often with a peribronchovascular and lower lobe predilection (**Fig. 8**).[103–105] The consolidation and ground-glass opacification is often admixed with traction bronchiectasis and reticulation, corresponding to a histologic pattern of OP on a background of fibrotic NSIP.[101,106,107] Indeed, the presence of pre-dominantly basal reticulation and ground-glass opacification, traction bronchiectasis, volume loss, and scattered bronchocentric foci of consolidation may be the radiologic clue to the diagnosis of an antisynthetase syndrome.[108] Foci of the perilobular pattern, a recognized manifestation of OP,[109] also may be seen.

There has been recent interest in the influence of different antibody profiles in DM and HRCT patterns. For instance, in clinically amyopathic dermatomyositis (CADM), the anti-CADM-140 antibody (recently renamed the anti-melanoma differentiation-associated gene 5 [anti-MDA5] antibody) is believed to be a factor in the development of ILD. Accordingly, in one small study, 12 of 25 patients with DM who were anti–CADM-140 positive, had significantly more lower-zone consolidation/ground-glass opacity and an absence of intralobular opacities than those who were negative for anti–CADM-140 (**Fig. 9**).[110] Hoshino and colleagues[111] also found a strikingly higher frequency of ILD in anti-MDA5–positive subjects as compared with those without anti-MDA5 antibodies (95% vs 32%, respectively) and there was a trend toward rapidly progressive lung disease. An interesting, but as yet unexplained, observation is the increased frequency of pneumomediastinum in patients with DM with a CADM phenotype,[112] especially in patients who are anti-MDA5 positive (see **Fig. 9**).[111]

### Sjögren syndrome

The prevalence of HRCT abnormalities in patients with SS with pulmonary symptoms has been estimated at 11%,[113] even though, somewhat counterintuitively, more than two-thirds of asymptomatic patients may demonstrate such abnormalities.[114] In SS, patients are more liable to develop impairment of upper respiratory tract immune defenses, glandular dysfunction, and bronchiolar inflammation, which probably explains why signs of airway involvement (ie, bronchial wall thickening, dilatation, and a mosaic attenuation pattern) are commonly seen.[115,116] The presence of airways disease

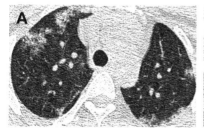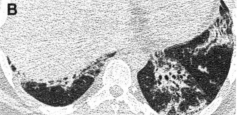

**Fig. 8.** A 31-year-old woman with a new diagnosis of polymyositis and anti-Jo1 antibody positivity. Transverse HRCT slices show patches of peripheral consolidation in the upper lobes (*A*) and more bronchocentric consolidation in the lower lobes (*B*), typical of the OP pattern seen in these patients.

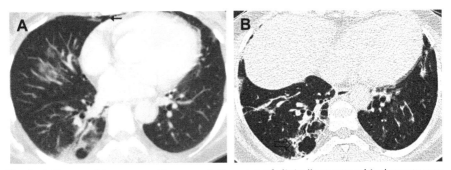

**Fig. 9.** A 50-year-old woman with a recent diagnosis of clinically amyopathic dermatomyositis and anti-MDA5 antibody positivity. (*A*) Transverse conventional (non–high-resolution) CT (2-mm slice thickness) demonstrates a bandlike opacity of consolidation in the apical segment of the right lower lobe, typical of OP. Note the pneumomediastinum (*arrow*), well-described in such patients. (*B*) Follow-up HRCT slice 3 months later shows persistence of consolidation in the right lower lobe, with the perilobular pattern of OP (*block arrow*) noted. The pneumomediastinum has resolved.

makes it difficult to gauge exactly how much of the parenchymal injury seen in SS is a consequence of airways-based inflammation, rather than a direct "hit" on the lung parenchyma. This notwithstanding, the ILD in SS is most commonly of an NSIP pattern, characterized by lower-zone ground-glass opacification and interlobular septal thickening.[117,118]

A pattern of lymphoid interstitial pneumonia (LIP) has been considered the commoner SS-associated ILD,[119,120] but it is possible that such statements were based on the subjective histologic interpretation of a homogeneous lymphocytic infiltrate as LIP rather than a cellular NSIP.[121] In some patients with LIP related to SS, HRCT may show patchy ground-glass opacities together with thin-walled parenchymal cysts, sometimes measuring up to 6 cm in diameter, as well as peribronchovascular, centrilobular, and subpleural nodules (**Fig. 10**).[114,117,118] The association among SS, LIP, and other lymphoproliferative disease is also worth remembering.[122] Indeed, the spectrum of lymphoproliferative disorder in SS varies and ranges from benign, as exemplified by the entity of follicular bronchiolitis (manifesting as a predominant

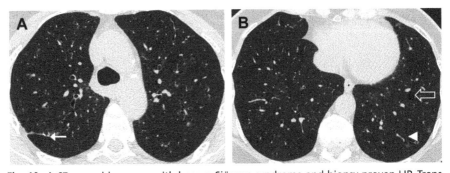

**Fig. 10.** A 67-year-old woman with known Sjögren syndrome and biopsy-proven LIP. Transverse HRCT slices show multiple foci of bronchocentric ground-glass opacity (*A*), as well as multiple thin-walled parenchymal cysts (*block arrow* in *B*). Traction bronchiectasis is present (*arrowhead* in *B*), concerning for an adverse prognosis. Note the surgical suture material postbiopsy in the posterior right upper lobe (*arrow* in *A*).

tree-in-bud pattern on HRCT),[116] to overt malignant lymphoma (usually of non-Hodgkin type). Lymphoma in patients with SS will present as nodules larger than 10 mm in diameter, foci of consolidation, mediastinal lymph node enlargement,[119,123] and pleural effusions.[123] A rare but striking presentation of LIP in SS occurs when there is associated pulmonary amyloid deposition; on HRCT there are multiple bizarrely shaped nodules (which may appear calcified) often adjacent to cysts, with no particular zonal predilection.[124–126]

### Mixed connective tissue disease

There is continuing debate about whether MCTD represents a distinct entity or a simply an "overlap syndrome" with features of, most commonly, SSc, SLE, and PM/DM.[127–129] There is support for the latter hypothesis in that the thoracic manifestations of MCTD generally represent an overlap of features found in the other CTDs listed previously. Lung disease, based on review of HRCT, is reported in more than 50% of patients with MCTD.[130,131] The most common abnormalities are reticulation and ground-glass opacification, which tend to be basal predominant and typically of limited extent (**Fig. 11**).[130–132] In one study, there was a reticular pattern at HRCT in just more than one-third of patients; in most cases, reticulation was admixed with fine intralobular lines or cysts measuring smaller than 4 mm in diameter.[130]

The reported prevalence of certain abnormalities in MCTD may differ from its "component" CTDs. In a rare direct comparison, Saito and colleagues[133] observed a lower frequency of ground-glass opacity in patients with MCTD compared with patients with SSc, SLE, and PM/DM, but found that interlobular septal thickening was present in all patients with MCTD, with an unexpectedly high proportion of honeycombing. A striking preponderance (98%) of subpleural nodularity also was noted in another study,[132] the reasons for which are unclear. Interestingly, although the clinical features of PM/DM may be present in patients with MCTD, the mixed NSIP-OP pattern described in PM/DM has, to the best of our knowledge, not been reported in MCTD. Other radiologic findings of MCTD-related thoracic disease include pleural thickening/effusions, esophageal dysmotility, centrilobular nodularity, and airway involvement, but are rare.

### Pulmonary Complications in Connective Tissue–Associated Disease

As discussed previously, the lung complications of CTDs are reasonably common. For practical purposes, these can be broadly thought of as acute and nonacute sequelae (**Table 3**). The imaging implications of these complications are reviewed in the following sections.

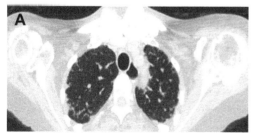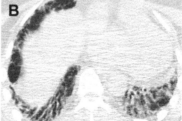

**Fig. 11.** A 52-year-old woman with MCTD with overlapping clinical features of SSc and RA. Transverse CT slice at the lung apices (*A*) demonstrates mild subpleural reticulation, in addition to the prominent dilated esophagus and marked soft tissue calcinosis surrounding the sternoclavicular and glenohumeral joints, while marked traction bronchiectasis and ground-glass opacity is seen at the bases (*B*), compatible with a fibrotic NSIP.

**Table 3**
**Complications and their relative frequencies in different connective tissue diseases**

| Complication | Connective Tissue Disease | | | | | |
|---|---|---|---|---|---|---|
| | RA | SSc | SLE | PM/DM | SS | MCTD |
| Acute | | | | | | |
|   Acute exacerbation | +++ | + | ++ | + | +++ | + |
|   Infection | +++ | + | ++ | + | + | ++ |
|   Pulmonary hemorrhage | + | + | +++[a] | + | + | + |
| Chronic | | | | | | |
|   Pulmonary hypertension | + | +++ | ++ | + | + | +++ |
|   Malignancy | ++ | + | ++ | +++[b] | ++ | + |

The number of + signs denotes the relative prevalence of the complication.

*Abbreviations:* MCTD, mixed connective tissue disease; PM/DM, polymyositis/dermatomyositis; RA, rheumatoid arthritis; SLE, systemic lupus erythematosus; SS, Sjögren syndrome; SSc, systemic sclerosis.

[a] Particularly associated with the antiphospholipid syndrome.
[b] PM/DM may represent a paraneoplastic manifestation of an underlying occult malignancy.

### Acute complications

When an abrupt clinical deterioration occurs in a patient with known CTD-associated lung disease, the clinician and radiologist must consider a number of possibilities. These will include the diagnosis of acute exacerbation of ILD, iatrogenic lung disease, opportunistic infection, and pulmonary hemorrhage.

Acute exacerbations, per se, are uncommon but statistically meaningful comparisons have been difficult because of the small study populations reported to date. Indeed, acute exacerbations are seen as the first presentation of an ILD in only a minority of cases. That said, patients with RA (**Fig. 12**) and primary SS seem to be at

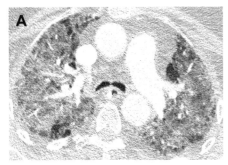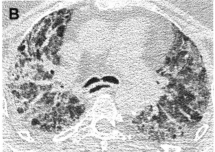

**Fig. 12.** Acute exacerbation of ILD in a 74-year-old woman with RA (same patient as in **Fig. 4**B) who had become significantly breathless after elective carotid endarterectomy. (A) Contrast-enhanced transverse CT slice at the level of the main PA shows diffuse ground-glass opacity with some fine reticulation, suggesting an alveolar infiltrate from DAD, but it is uncertain whether this is being exaggerated by the combined effect of iodinated contrast and a predominantly expiratory CT (note the narrow caliber of the right and left main bronchi proximally), or indeed if an element of alveolar edema is present. (B) Transverse unenhanced HRCT at the same level only 10 days later demonstrates that the pattern of predominant ground-glass opacity has evolved into predominantly coarse reticulation and patchy consolidation, concerning for the organizing phase of a DAD in the context of an acute exacerbation.

highest risk of acute exacerbation.[134–136] Acute deterioration also is recognized in SLE ("lupus pneumonitis") with earlier studies suggesting a prevalence of 2% to 9%,[83,137–139] although one series (consisting solely of patients with SLE) reported this as the presenting manifestation in as many as 50%.[140] The outlook for patients with RA with acute exacerbation is generally poorer with increasing age,[134,141] and in those with a known preexisting ILD.[135] There are conflicting reports on whether the survival of patients with RA with such exacerbations is worse in the presence of a UIP pattern.[48,141] Regardless of the underlying CTD, the histologic hallmark of acute exacerbations is diffuse alveolar damage (DAD). As an aside, the term acute interstitial pneumonia (AIP) has occasionally been used to denote any interstitial pneumonia of acute onset, including acute exacerbations of IIP, and is characterized histologically by DAD as well. However, AIP should be strictly reserved for acute rapidly progressive dyspnea due to interstitial disease without an identified cause.[8]

Drug toxicity in patients with CTD typically arises from treatment with methotrexate and leflunomide: the quoted toxicity rates are 0.3% to 11.0%[142,143] and 1.0%,[144,145] respectively. Interestingly, a recent prospective study found that when HRCT data were integrated with the application of stringent criteria for a diagnosis of methotrexate-induced drug toxicity (ie, radiologic improvement after drug cessation and a clinical course consistent with a hypersensitivity reaction), the prevalence of methotrexate toxicity was only 1%.[146] At this point, it is important to note that the histologic patterns of pulmonary injury are not specific to any particular drug. Indeed, in cases in which biopsy has been undertaken, the pathologist may expect to encounter a spectrum of histopathologic patterns, including DAD, OP, hypersensitivity pneumonitis, and pulmonary hemorrhage, as well as pulmonary edema caused by cardiac toxicity.

Diffuse alveolar hemorrhage (DAH) can complicate the clinical and radiologic picture, especially in SLE.[147,148] Radiographically, DAH manifests as airspace and/or interstitial infiltrates that may be diffuse, basal, or perihilar in distribution, and is often bilateral.[148,149] Pleural effusions are not infrequent, being reported in 27% of episodes in one study.[150] On HRCT, patchy centrilobular nodules (representing conglomerations of hemosiderin-laden macrophages within alveoli) with no zonal predilection and ground-glass opacities are seen (**Fig. 13**)[151]; a "crazy-paving" pattern (a

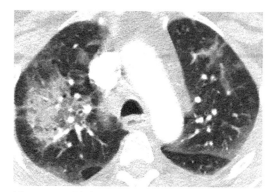

**Fig. 13.** A 46-year-old woman with known SLE and antiphospholipid syndrome, presenting with 12 hours of hemoptysis. Contrast-enhanced CT demonstrates patchy ground-glass opacity likely representing pulmonary hemorrhage. However, such an appearance can be indistinguishable from DAD, atypical infection, or a lymphoproliferative disorder, and interpretation relies on clinical context and evolution on serial imaging.

combination of ground-glass opacification and interlobular septal thickening) has rarely been reported.[152]

Opportunistic infections may be problematic in patients with CTDs and contribute to both morbidity and mortality.[153] Of note, there is a predisposition to mycobacterial infections with the increased use of tumor necrosis factor inhibitors.[154–156] Patients with CTD also may develop *Pneumocystis jiroveci* pneumonia (PCP), primarily as a consequence of long-term immunosuppressive therapy.[157]

Distinguishing between the acute pulmonary complications described previously on imaging tests can be challenging. For instance, the presence of a histologic pattern of DAD (whether associated with acute exacerbation, caused by drug toxicity, or even as a systemic inflammatory response to infection), will only ever manifest with diffuse bilateral airspace opacification, with variably extensive ground-glass opacification, admixed reticulation (with or without traction bronchiectasis) and foci of consolidation.[43,134,135,158] These features are similar to acute DAD occurring in other clinical contexts.[159–162] In the absence of any consolidation, the pattern of DAD on HRCT may be impossible to distinguish from pulmonary hemorrhage, opportunistic PCP and pulmonary edema. The presence of pleural fluid might push the radiologist to consider coexistent cardiac dysfunction, but, because pleural effusions are also a feature of acute decline (particularly in SLE), the differential diagnosis of acute exacerbation would still need to be entertained. The presence of centrilobular or subpleural micronodules might suggest an element of subacute hypersensitivity pneumonitis,[163,164] but these also are a feature of pulmonary hypertension in some patients (as discussed in the next section).

### Nonacute complications

Pulmonary hypertension (PH) is perhaps the most serious of the nonacute complications of CTDs and is most problematic in patients with SSc and MCTD.[165] PH has an estimated prevalence in SSc, MCTD, and SLE of 10% to 16%,[166–168] 10% to 45%,[169] and 4%,[170] respectively. Interestingly, although the overall prevalence of PH is higher in the presence of ILD, the severity of PH may be disproportionately greater than expected for the often limited ILD extent encountered in SSc[171]; this probably reflects the contribution of vasculopathy in the microcirculation to raised pulmonary vascular resistance, a phenomenon that is not immediately obvious on conventional HRCT.

On HRCT, PH is suspected when there is an increase in the transverse diameter of the main pulmonary artery (PA), as seen at the level of its bifurcation: a diameter greater than 2.9 cm[172] or, alternatively, an increase in the ratio of diameters of the main PA to ascending aorta (AA) higher than 1 (**Fig. 14**)[173] has been considered predictive of raised PA pressure. However, the absolute measurement of PA is probably an unreliable marker of PH in the presence of pulmonary fibrosis (from any cause), whereas the usefulness of the PA/AA ratio appears to be preserved.[174] Against this, it is should be noted that the value of the PA/AA ratio has not been studied in CTD-ILD populations exclusively. An occasional feature of PH is centrilobular nodules, corresponding histopathologically to cholesterol granulomas.[175] Pleural effusions may occur in just fewer than 40%,[176] but the mechanism for its occurrence in PH is not clear.

A final mention should be made of the increased risk of malignancy in all CTDs.[177–182] The risk of lymphoma (particularly primary pulmonary lymphomas) is higher in RA, SS, and SLE.[181,183] In patients with PM/DM, the CTD may be a paraneoplastic manifestation of an underlying malignancy.[184] An underlying malignancy should thus always be considered in the differential diagnosis of nonresolving airspace opacity or enlarged/enlarging thoracic lymph nodes.

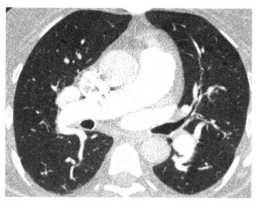

**Fig. 14.** A 59-year-old woman with SLE and known antiphospholipid syndrome and PH confirmed on right heart catheterization. Transverse contrast-enhanced CT slice at the level of the main PA demonstrates an enlarged main PA (3.1 cm), but also markedly enlarged and tortuous segmental PAs, suspicious for PH.

## THE ROLE OF HIGH-RESOLUTION COMPUTED TOMOGRAPHY IN DIAGNOSTIC EVALUATION, MONITORING, AND PROGNOSTICATION

In CTD-related ILD, HRCT may have a role in monitoring patients with established lung disease, identifying complications, evaluating treatment response, and predicting outcome.

In monitoring CTD-ILD, serial HRCT may show progression in the extent of fibrosis. However, trends in pulmonary function tests (PFTs) and clinical behavior are probably as informative when there has been deterioration in HRCT appearances. For instance, Moore and colleagues[185] recently showed that in a cohort of patients with SSc followed for a mean of 3.5 years, patients who demonstrated a substantial deterioration in their HRCT ILD abnormalities had a correspondingly detectable decline of at least 30% in forced vital capacity (FVC), DLco, or DLco corrected for alveolar volume. For this reason, routine serial HRCT for disease monitoring may not be necessary. However, HRCT may play an important role in complementing functional assessment when physiologic decline is not easily attributable solely to ILD, for instance, in the setting of SSc-related pulmonary vasculopathy in SSc, or progressive bronchiolitis obliterans in RA.

Earlier evidence suggests that the pattern of fibrosis on HRCT is unlikely to predict response to treatment.[186] However, Roth and colleagues[107] recently showed that patients with SSc who demonstrate a reticular pattern, occupying at least half of any of the 3 lung zones (upper, mid, and lower) as determined on HRCT, are more likely to respond to treatment. Conversely, HRCT also may have a role when trying to assess which patients may potentially suffer drug-related pulmonary toxicity. In one series, 57% of asymptomatic patients with RA and ILD abnormalities seen on HRCT demonstrated a tendency toward progressive ILD abnormalities, and this tendency was significantly related to higher frequencies of methotrexate treatment.[54]

Several outcome studies, specifically in the setting of CTD-related fibrotic lung disease, have involved analysis of multiple variables, including HRCT pattern scores, PFTs, and clinical data. The morphologic severity of fibrosis, assessed by HRCT, and physiologic severity, assessed by lung function (in particular DLco), have been shown to independently predict survival, raising the possibility that more powerful prognostic discrimination may be expected from an integration of both.[18,21] Management decisions in ILD tend to be based on outcomes that are dichotomous. For example, is the patient likely to respond to treatment or not? Therefore, "staging" patients by separating them into 2 prognostic categories (such as good prognosis/poor prognosis or limited disease/extensive disease) to answer these dichotomous decisions is desirable. This dichotomous approach has been applied to SSc-related ILD, using a simple staging system for rapid stratification of clinical risk (**Fig. 15**).[188] By separating patients into 1 of 2 prognostically distinct categories, patients who may benefit from treatment may be more readily separated from those who are likely to progress regardless of treatment. First, an evaluation of global interstitial disease extent on HRCT with respect to a threshold of 20% is made. Patients whose global interstitial disease extent is considered indeterminate (ie, close to the 20% threshold) are then evaluated based on their percent-predicted FVC for which a threshold of 70% is used. In this way, patients are categorized into 2 groups, namely "limited" or "extensive" disease, which are strikingly prognostically distinct. The strengths of this system are twofold: first, by combining HRCT and pulmonary function, a stronger prognostic discrimination is obtained than that provided by either of the 2 variables in isolation. Second, the staging model allows for instances in which the HRCT data are marginal (ie, global disease extent very close to 20%) by providing recourse to a threshold for FVC. This is an important advantage, as it means that all patients may be categorized regardless of the clinician's experience in evaluating HRCT.

The overlap of clinical and ILD phenotypes in CTD-ILD may pose a particular problem, as it somewhat prevents the generalization of prognostic HRCT data from one type of CTD to CTDs at large. To circumvent this limitation, Walsh and colleagues[18] studied the prognostic discrimination provided by HRCT, as well as PFT data, in an "all-comers" cohort of patients with CTD-ILD. On multivariate analysis, they demonstrated that traction bronchiectasis (either measured semiquantitatively or using a binary "absence or presence" score) and extent of honeycombing (both prognostic indicators in IIPs),[189] as well as DLco, were independently associated with increased mortality. Furthermore, in a subset of patients with surgical biopsy data, it was shown

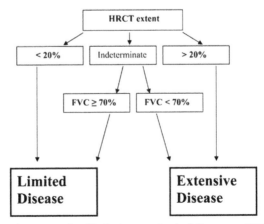

**Fig. 15.** A simple staging system for SSc that uses extent of disease on HRCT and PFTs to separate patients into 2 prognostically distinct groups. (*From* Goh NS, Desai SR, Veeraraghavan S, et al. Interstitial lung disease in systemic sclerosis: a simple staging system. Am J Respir Crit Care Med 2008;177:1249; with permission.)

that a radiologic-pathologic concordance with respect to diagnosis influenced survival. Patients with a radiologic diagnosis of fibrotic NSIP but histopathologic evidence of UIP had a more favorable outcome when compared with patients whose radiologic and histopathologic appearances suggested UIP. The latter finding makes a possible case for surgical biopsy to provide additional prognostic information in the setting of a non-UIP pattern on HRCT, but such decisions would always need to be made on a case-by-case basis.

The prognostic studies by Goh and colleagues[188] and Walsh and colleagues[18] are perhaps even more pertinent because they provide simple reproducible systems for prognostication, with good interobserver agreement, that are easily replicated.[185] However, prospective studies on prognostication are still lacking to validate these methods.

## HIGH-RESOLUTION COMPUTED TOMOGRAPHY IN THE MULTIDISCIPLINARY WORKUP OF INTERSTITIAL LUNG DISEASE WITH NO PREVIOUS CONNECTIVE TISSUE DISEASE DIAGNOSIS

It has been estimated that 15% of patients presenting with IIP may have an underlying CTD,[190] and that 21% of apparently idiopathic NSIP and 13% of patients with IPF could be classifiable as an undifferentiated CTD.[191] Several descriptions of patients with autoantibodies suggestive of, but not diagnostic for, an underlying CTD have been published in recent years,[93,108,192,193] highlighting the importance of multidisciplinary evaluation of these patients. The concept of a "lung-dominant" CTD as proposed by Fischer and colleagues[194] and interstitial pneumonia with autoimmune features to denote ILD where there is a suspicion of a connective tissue disorder, have been suggested. In the authors' experience, patients referred for ILD workup are best evaluated by a multidisciplinary team that includes rheumatological expertise (**Fig. 16**). It is worth highlighting the importance of not mislabeling patients as having

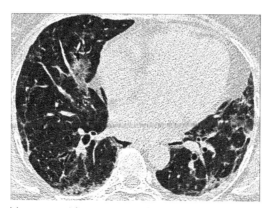

**Fig. 16.** A 55-year-old woman with recent-onset breathlessness, who had been given a diagnosis of IPF. When assessed in a joint rheumatology–diffuse lung disease clinic, she described experiencing some muscle weakness and joint pains over the preceding 4 months, and serology was positive for anti-Jo1 antibody. Although she did not satisfy all diagnostic criteria for polymyositis, the HRCT findings of subpleural ground-glass opacity, peripheral consolidation, and a perilobular pattern are consistent with the mixed NSIP-OP pattern seen in antisynthetase syndrome. The patient was therefore considered to have a lung-dominant connective tissue disease, and her symptoms successfully ameliorated with immunosuppression.

idiopathic ILD (and therefore limiting therapeutic options) when an undeclared CTD may be present.

## SUMMARY

The imaging features of the pulmonary manifestations of rheumatological disease and their pathologic and functional correlations have been progressively characterized over the past 3 decades. The interpretation of these images requires a methodical approach incorporating pattern recognition, appraisal of the extents of various component interstitial and airspace abnormalities, and awareness of prognostic signs, as well as an understanding of the pulmonary complications that occur in these disease entities. As the multidisciplinary approach to diagnosing and treating these diseases evolves, the role of imaging in both research and clinical interpretation of these diverse and challenging conditions will doubtless only continue to grow.

## REFERENCES

1. Epler GR, McLoud TC, Gaensler EA, et al. Normal chest roentgenograms in chronic diffuse infiltrative lung disease. N Engl J Med 1978;298:934–9.
2. Mathieson JR, Mayo JR, Staples CA, et al. Chronic diffuse infiltrative lung disease: comparison of diagnostic accuracy of CT and chest radiography. Radiology 1989;171:111–6.
3. Gabbay E, Tarala R, Will R, et al. Interstitial lung disease in recent onset rheumatoid arthritis. Am J Respir Crit Care Med 1997;156:528–35.
4. Schurawitzki H, Stiglbauer R, Graninger W, et al. Interstitial lung disease in progressive systemic sclerosis: high-resolution CT versus radiography. Radiology 1990;176:755–9.
5. Sant SM, Doran M, Fenelon HM, et al. Pleuropulmonary abnormalities in patients with systemic lupus erythematosus: assessment with high resolution computed tomography, chest radiography and pulmonary function tests. Clin Exp Rheumatol 1997;15:507–13.
6. American Thoracic Society, European Respiratory Society. American Thoracic Society/European Respiratory Society International Multidisciplinary Consensus Classification of the Idiopathic Interstitial Pneumonias. This joint statement of the American Thoracic Society (ATS), and the European Respiratory Society (ERS) was adopted by the ATS board of directors, June 2001 and by the ERS Executive Committee, June 2001. Am J Respir Crit Care Med 2002;165:277–304.
7. Raghu G, Collard HR, Egan JJ, et al. An official ATS/ERS/JRS/ALAT statement: idiopathic pulmonary fibrosis: evidence-based guidelines for diagnosis and management. Am J Respir Crit Care Med 2011;183:788–824.
8. Travis WD, Costabel U, Hansell DM, et al. An official American Thoracic Society/European Respiratory Society statement: update of the international multidisciplinary classification of the idiopathic interstitial pneumonias. Am J Respir Crit Care Med 2013;188:733–48.
9. Hartman TE, Swensen SJ, Hansell DM, et al. Nonspecific interstitial pneumonia: variable appearance at high-resolution chest CT. Radiology 2000;217:701–5.
10. Sverzellati N, Wells AU, Tomassetti S, et al. Biopsy-proved idiopathic pulmonary fibrosis: spectrum of nondiagnostic thin-section CT diagnoses. Radiology 2010; 254:957–64.
11. Sumikawa H, Johkoh T, Fujimoto K, et al. Pathologically proved nonspecific interstitial pneumonia: CT pattern analysis as compared with usual interstitial pneumonia CT pattern. Radiology 2014;272:549–56.

12. Johkoh T, Muller NL, Cartier Y, et al. Idiopathic interstitial pneumonias: diagnostic accuracy of thin-section CT in 129 patients. Radiology 1999;211: 555–60.

13. Lynch DA, Godwin JD, Safrin S, et al. High-resolution computed tomography in idiopathic pulmonary fibrosis: diagnosis and prognosis. Am J Respir Crit Care Med 2005;172:488–93.

14. Elliot TL, Lynch DA, Newell JD, et al. High-resolution computed tomography features of nonspecific interstitial pneumonia and usual interstitial pneumonia. J Comput Assist Tomogr 2005;29:339–45.

15. MacDonald SL, Rubens MB, Hansell DM, et al. Non-specific interstitial pneumonia and usual interstitial pneumonia: comparative appearances at and diagnostic accuracy of thin-section CT. Radiology 2001;221:600–5.

16. Watadani T, Sakai F, Johkoh T, et al. Interobserver variability in the CT assessment of honeycombing in the lungs. Radiology 2013;266:936–44.

17. Goldin JG, Lynch DA, Strollo DC, et al. High-resolution CT scan findings in patients with symptomatic scleroderma-related interstitial lung disease. Chest 2008;134:358–67.

18. Walsh SL, Sverzellati N, Devaraj A, et al. Connective tissue disease related fibrotic lung disease: high resolution computed tomographic and pulmonary function indices as prognostic determinants. Thorax 2014;69:216–22.

19. Johkoh T, Sakai F, Noma S, et al. Honeycombing on CT; its definition, pathologic correlation, and future direction of its diagnosis. Eur J Radiol 2014;83:27–31.

20. Tanaka N, Kim JS, Newell JD, et al. Rheumatoid arthritis-related lung diseases: CT findings. Radiology 2004;232:81–91.

21. Kim EJ, Elicker BM, Maldonado F, et al. Usual interstitial pneumonia in rheumatoid arthritis-associated interstitial lung disease. Eur Respir J 2010;35:1322–8.

22. Tansey D, Wells AU, Colby TV, et al. Variations in histological patterns of interstitial pneumonia between connective tissue disorders and their relationship to prognosis. Histopathology 2004;44:585–96.

23. Bouros D, Wells AU, Nicholson AG, et al. Histopathologic subsets of fibrosing alveolitis in patients with systemic sclerosis and their relationship to outcome. Am J Respir Crit Care Med 2002;165:1581–6.

24. Hwang JH, Misumi S, Sahin H, et al. Computed tomographic features of idiopathic fibrosing interstitial pneumonia: comparison with pulmonary fibrosis related to collagen vascular disease. J Comput Assist Tomogr 2009;33:410–5.

25. Muller NL, Staples CA, Miller RR, et al. Disease activity in idiopathic pulmonary fibrosis: CT and pathologic correlation. Radiology 1987;165:731–4.

26. Wells AU, Hansell DM, Rubens MB, et al. The predictive value of appearances on thin-section computed tomography in fibrosing alveolitis. Am Rev Respir Dis 1993;148:1076–82.

27. Wells AU, Rubens MB, du Bois RM, et al. Serial CT in fibrosing alveolitis: prognostic significance of the initial pattern. AJR Am J Roentgenol 1993;161: 1159–65.

28. Silva CI, Muller NL, Hansell DM, et al. Nonspecific interstitial pneumonia and idiopathic pulmonary fibrosis: changes in pattern and distribution of disease over time. Radiology 2008;247:251–9.

29. Hartman TE, Primack SL, Kang EY, et al. Disease progression in usual interstitial pneumonia compared with desquamative interstitial pneumonia. Assessment with serial CT. Chest 1996;110:378–82.

30. Wells AU, Hansell DM, Corrin B, et al. High resolution computed tomography as a predictor of lung histology in systemic sclerosis. Thorax 1992;47:738–42.

31. Dawson JK, Fewins HE, Desmond J, et al. Fibrosing alveolitis in patients with rheumatoid arthritis as assessed by high resolution computed tomography, chest radiography, and pulmonary function tests. Thorax 2001;56: 622–7.

32. Remy-Jardin M, Giraud F, Remy J, et al. Importance of ground-glass attenuation in chronic diffuse infiltrative lung disease: pathologic-CT correlation. Radiology 1993;189:693–8.

33. Ellman P, Ball RE. Rheumatoid disease with joint and pulmonary manifestations. Br Med J 1948;2:816–20.

34. Olson AL, Swigris JJ, Sprunger DB, et al. Rheumatoid arthritis-interstitial lung disease-associated mortality. Am J Respir Crit Care Med 2011;183:372–8.

35. Bongartz T, Nannini C, Medina-Velasquez YF, et al. Incidence and mortality of interstitial lung disease in rheumatoid arthritis: a population-based study. Arthritis Rheum 2010;62:1583–91.

36. Biederer J, Schnabel A, Muhle C, et al. Correlation between HRCT findings, pulmonary function tests and bronchoalveolar lavage cytology in interstitial lung disease associated with rheumatoid arthritis. Eur Radiol 2004;14:272–80.

37. Hassan WU, Keaney NP, Holland CD, et al. High resolution computed tomography of the lung in lifelong non-smoking patients with rheumatoid arthritis. Ann Rheum Dis 1995;54:308–10.

38. Remy-Jardin M, Remy J, Cortet B, et al. Lung changes in rheumatoid arthritis: CT findings. Radiology 1994;193:375–82.

39. Hillarby MC, McMahon MJ, Grennan DM, et al. HLA associations in subjects with rheumatoid arthritis and bronchiectasis but not with other pulmonary complications of rheumatoid disease. Br J Rheumatol 1993;32:794–7.

40. Perez T, Remy-Jardin M, Cortet B. Airways involvement in rheumatoid arthritis: clinical, functional, and HRCT findings. Am J Respir Crit Care Med 1998;157: 1658–65.

41. Cortet B, Perez T, Roux N, et al. Pulmonary function tests and high resolution computed tomography of the lungs in patients with rheumatoid arthritis. Ann Rheum Dis 1997;56:596–600.

42. Devouassoux G, Cottin V, Lioté H, et al. Characterisation of severe obliterative bronchiolitis in rheumatoid arthritis. Eur Respir J 2009;33:1053–61.

43. Akira M, Sakatani M, Hara H. Thin-section CT findings in rheumatoid arthritis-associated lung disease: CT patterns and their courses. J Comput Assist Tomogr 1999;23:941–8.

44. Nakamura Y, Suda T, Kaida Y, et al. Rheumatoid lung disease: prognostic analysis of 54 biopsy-proven cases. Respir Med 2012;106:1164–9.

45. Wilsher M, Voight L, Milne D, et al. Prevalence of airway and parenchymal abnormalities in newly diagnosed rheumatoid arthritis. Respir Med 2012;106: 1441–6.

46. Mori S, Isamu C, Koga Y, et al. Comparison of pulmonary abnormalities on high-resolution computed tomography in patients with early versus long-standing rheumatoid arthritis. J Rheumatol 2008;35:1513–20.

47. Howling SJ, Hansell DM, Wells AU, et al. Follicular bronchiolitis: thin-section CT and histologic findings. Radiology 1999;212:637–42.

48. Tsuchiya Y, Takayanagi N, Sugiura H, et al. Lung diseases directly associated with rheumatoid arthritis and their relationship to outcome. Eur Respir J 2011; 37:1411–7.

49. Hayakawa H, Sato A, Imokawa S, et al. Bronchiolar disease in rheumatoid arthritis. Am J Respir Crit Care Med 1996;154:1531–6.

50. Geddes DM, Corrin B, Brewerton DA, et al. Progressive airway obliteration in adults and its association with rheumatoid disease. Q J Med 1977;184:427–44.
51. Yoshinouchi T, Ohtsuki Y, Fujita J, et al. Nonspecific interstitial pneumonia pattern as pulmonary involvement of rheumatoid arthritis. Rheumatol Int 2005; 26:121–5.
52. Lee HK, Kim DS, Yoo B, et al. Histopathologic pattern and clinical features of rheumatoid arthritis-associated interstitial lung disease. Chest 2005;127:2019–27.
53. Assayag D, Elicker BM, Urbania TH, et al. Rheumatoid arthritis-associated interstitial lung disease: radiologic identification of usual interstitial pneumonia pattern. Radiology 2014;270:583–8.
54. Gochuico BR, Avila NA, Chow CK, et al. Progressive preclinical interstitial lung disease in rheumatoid arthritis. Arch Intern Med 2008;168:159–66.
55. Doyle TJ, Dellaripa PF, Batra K, et al. Functional impact of a spectrum of interstitial lung abnormalities in rheumatoid arthritis. Chest 2014;146:41–50.
56. Assayag D, Lubin M, Lee JS, et al. Predictors of mortality in rheumatoid arthritis-related interstitial lung disease. Respirology 2014;19:493–500.
57. Kelly CA, Saravanan V, Nisar M, et al. Rheumatoid arthritis-related interstitial lung disease: associations, prognostic factors and physiological and radiological characteristics—a large multicentre UK study. Rheumatology (Oxford) 2014;53:1676–82.
58. Antoniou KM, Walsh SL, Hansell DM, et al. Smoking-related emphysema is associated with idiopathic pulmonary fibrosis and rheumatoid lung. Respirology 2013;18:1191–6.
59. Mori S, Koga Y, Sugimoto M. Different risk factors between interstitial lung disease and airway disease in rheumatoid arthritis. Respir Med 2012;106:1591–9.
60. Yousem SA, Colby TV, Carrington CB. Lung biopsy in rheumatoid arthritis. Am Rev Respir Dis 1985;131:770–7.
61. Sahn SA. Immunologic diseases of the pleura. Clin Chest Med 1985;6:83–102.
62. Remy-Jardin M, Remy J, Wallaert B, et al. Pulmonary involvement in progressive systemic sclerosis: sequential evaluation with CT, pulmonary function tests, and bronchoalveolar lavage. Radiology 1993;188:499–506.
63. Devenyi K, Czirjak L. High resolution computed tomography for the evaluation of lung involvement in 101 patients with scleroderma. Clin Rheumatol 1995;14: 633–40.
64. Arroliga AC, Podell DN, Matthay RA. Pulmonary manifestations of scleroderma. J Thorac Imaging 1992;7:30–45.
65. Desai SR, Veeraraghavan S, Hansell DM, et al. CT features of lung disease in patients with systemic sclerosis: comparison with idiopathic pulmonary fibrosis and non-specific interstitial pneumonia. Radiology 2004;232:560–7.
66. Kim DS, Yoo B, Lee JS, et al. The major histopathologic pattern of pulmonary fibrosis in scleroderma is nonspecific interstitial pneumonia. Sarcoidosis Vasc Diffuse Lung Dis 2002;19:121–7.
67. Muir TE, Tazelaar HD, Colby TV, et al. Organizing diffuse alveolar damage associated with progressive systemic sclerosis. Mayo Clin Proc 1997;72:639–42.
68. Bridges AJ, Hsu KC, Dias-Arias AA, et al. Bronchiolitis obliterans organizing pneumonia and scleroderma. J Rheumatol 1992;19:1136–40.
69. Tashkin DP, Elashoff R, Clements PJ, et al. Cyclophosphamide versus placebo in scleroderma lung disease. N Engl J Med 2006;354:2655–66.
70. De Santis M, Bosello S, La Torre G, et al. Functional, radiological and biological markers of alveolitis and infections of the lower respiratory tract in patients with systemic sclerosis. Respir Res 2005;6:96.

71. Launay D, Remy-Jardin M, Michon-Pasturel U, et al. High resolution computed tomography in fibrosing alveolitis associated with systemic sclerosis. J Rheumatol 2006;33:1789–801.

72. Kim EA, Johkoh T, Lee KS, et al. Interstitial pneumonia in progressive systemic sclerosis: serial high-resolution CT findings with functional correlation. J Comput Assist Tomogr 2001;25:757–63.

73. Shah RM, Jimenez S, Wechsler R. Significance of ground-glass opacity on HRCT in long-term follow-up of patients with systemic sclerosis. J Thorac Imaging 2007;22:120–4.

74. Warrick JH, Bhalla M, Schabel SI, et al. High resolution computed tomography in early scleroderma lung disease. J Rheumatol 1991;18:1520–8.

75. Bhalla M, Silver RM, Shepard JA, et al. Chest CT in patients with scleroderma: prevalence of asymptomatic esophageal dilatation and mediastinal lymphadenopathy. AJR Am J Roentgenol 1993;161:269–72.

76. Chan TY, Hansell DM, Rubens MB, et al. Cryptogenic fibrosing alveolitis and the fibrosing alveolitis of systemic sclerosis: morphological differences on computed tomographic scans. Thorax 1997;52:265–70.

77. Abu-Shakra M, Guillemin F, Lee P. Gastrointestinal manifestations of systemic sclerosis. Semin Arthritis Rheum 1994;24:29–39.

78. Vonk MC, van Die CE, Snoeren MM, et al. Oesophageal dilatation on high-resolution computed tomography scan of the lungs as a sign of scleroderma. Ann Rheum Dis 2008;67:1317–21.

79. Christmann RB, Wells AU, Capelozzi VL, et al. Gastroesophageal reflux incites interstitial lung disease in systemic sclerosis: clinical, radiologic, histopathologic, and treatment evidence. Semin Arthritis Rheum 2010;40:241–9.

80. Marie I, Dominique S, Levesque H, et al. Esophageal involvement and pulmonary manifestations in systemic sclerosis. Arthritis Rheum 2001;45:346–54.

81. Gilson M, Zerkak D, Wipff J, et al. Prognostic factors for lung function in systemic sclerosis: prospective study of 105 cases. Eur Respir J 2010;35:112–7.

82. D'Angelo WA, Fries JF, Masi AT, et al. Pathologic observations in systemic sclerosis (scleroderma). A study of fifty-eight autopsy cases and fifty-eight matched controls. Am J Med 1969;46:428–40.

83. Kim JS, Lee KS, Koh EM, et al. Thoracic involvement of systemic lupus erythematosus: clinical, pathologic, and radiologic findings. J Comput Assist Tomogr 2000;24:9–18.

84. Wiedemann HP, Matthay RA. Pulmonary manifestations of systemic lupus erythematosus. J Thorac Imaging 1992;7:1–18.

85. Orens JB, Martinez FJ, Lynch JP III. Pleuropulmonary manifestations of systemic lupus erythematosus. Rheum Dis Clin North Am 1994;20:159–93.

86. Fenlon HM, Doran M, Sant SM, et al. High-resolution chest CT in systemic lupus erythematosus. AJR Am J Roentgenol 1996;166:301–7.

87. Ooi GC, Ngan H, Peh WC, et al. Systemic lupus erythematosus patients with respiratory symptoms: the value of HRCT. Clin Radiol 1997;52:775–81.

88. Weinrib L, Sharma OP, Quismorio FP. A long-term study of interstitial lung disease in systemic lupus erythematosus. Semin Arthritis Rheum 1990;20:48–56.

89. Jacobsen S, Petersen J, Ullman S, et al. A multicentre study of 513 Danish patients with systemic lupus erythematosus. I. Disease manifestations and analyses of clinical subsets. Clin Rheumatol 1998;17:468–77.

90. Oki H, Aoki T, Saito K, et al. Thin-section chest CT findings in systemic lupus erythematosus with antiphospholipid syndrome: a comparison with systemic

lupus erythematosus without antiphospholipid syndrome. Eur J Radiol 2012;81: 1335–9.

91. Hoffbrand BI, Beck ER. "Unexplained" dyspnoea and shrinking lungs in systemic lupus erythematosus. Br Med J 1965;1:1273–7.

92. Thompson PJ, Dhillon DP, Ledingham J, et al. Shrinking lungs, diaphragmatic dysfunction, and systemic lupus erythematosus. Am Rev Respir Dis 1985;132: 926–8.

93. Allen D, Fischer A, Bshouty Z, et al. Evaluating systemic lupus erythematosus patients for lung involvement. Lupus 2012;21:1316–25.

94. Gibson CJ, Edmonds JP, Hughes GR. Diaphragm function and lung involvement in systemic lupus erythematosus. Am J Med 1977;63:926–32.

95. Martens J, Demedts M, Vanmeenen MT, et al. Respiratory muscle dysfunction in systemic lupus erythematosus. Chest 1983;84:170–5.

96. Laroche CM, Mulvey DA, Hawkins PN, et al. Diaphragm strength in the shrinking lung syndrome of systemic lupus erythematosus. Q J Med 1989;71:429–39.

97. Hawkins P, Davison AG, Dasgupta B, et al. Diaphragm strength in acute systemic lupus erythematosus in a patient with paradoxical abdominal motion and reduced lung volumes. Thorax 2001;56:329–30.

98. Betteridge Z, Gunawardena H, North J, et al. Anti-synthetase syndrome: a new autoantibody to phenylalanyl transfer RNA synthetase (anti-Zo) associated with polymyositis and interstitial pneumonia. Rheumatology (Oxford) 2007;46:1005–8.

99. Gunawardena H, Betteridge ZE, McHugh NJ. Myositis-specific autoantibodies: their clinical and pathogenic significance in disease expression. Rheumatology (Oxford) 2009;48:607–12.

100. Schmidt WA, Wetzel W, Friedlander R, et al. Clinical and serological aspects of patients with anti-Jo-1 antibodies—an evolving spectrum of disease manifestations. Clin Rheumatol 2000;19:371–7.

101. Mileti LM, Strek ME, Niewold TB, et al. Clinical characteristics of patients with anti-Jo-1 antibodies: a single center experience. J Clin Rheumatol 2009;15:254–5.

102. Vancsa A, Csipo I, Nemeth J, et al. Characteristics of interstitial lung disease in SS-A positive/Jo-1 positive inflammatory myopathy patients. Rheumatol Int 2009;29:989–94.

103. Bonnefoy O, Ferretti G, Calaque O, et al. Serial chest CT findings in interstitial lung disease associated with polymyositis-dermatomyositis. Eur J Radiol 2004;49:235–44.

104. Fathi M, Vikgren J, Boijsen M, et al. Interstitial lung disease in polymyositis and dermatomyositis: longitudinal evaluation by pulmonary function and radiology. Arthritis Rheum 2008;59:677–85.

105. Ikezoe J, Johkoh T, Kohno N, et al. High-resolution CT findings of lung disease in patients with polymyositis and dermatomyositis. J Thorac Imaging 1996;11: 250–9.

106. Richards TJ, Eggebeen A, Gibson K, et al. Characterization and peripheral blood biomarker assessment of anti-Jo-1 antibody-positive interstitial lung disease. Arthritis Rheum 2009;60:2183–92.

107. Ingegnoli F, Lubatti C, Ingegnoli A, et al. Interstitial lung disease outcomes by high-resolution computed tomography (HRCT) in anti-Jo1 antibody-positive polymyositis patients: a single centre study and review of the literature. Autoimmun Rev 2012;11:335–40.

108. Fischer A, Swigris JJ, du Bois RM, et al. Anti-synthetase syndrome in ANA and anti-Jo-1 negative patients presenting with idiopathic interstitial pneumonia. Respir Med 2009;103:1719–24.

109. Ujita M, Renzoni EA, Veeraraghavan S, et al. Organizing pneumonia: perilobular pattern at thin-section CT. Radiology 2004;232:757–61.

110. Tanizawa K, Handa T, Nakashima R, et al. HRCT features of interstitial lung disease in dermatomyositis with anti-CADM-140 antibody. Respir Med 2011;105: 1380–7.

111. Hoshino K, Muro Y, Sugiura K, et al. Anti-MDA5 and anti-TIF1-gamma antibodies have clinical significance for patients with dermatomyositis. Rheumatology (Oxford) 2010;49:1726–33.

112. Le Goff B, Cherin P, Cantagrel A, et al. Pneumomediastinum in interstitial lung disease associated with dermatomyositis and polymyositis. Arthritis Rheum 2009;61:108–18.

113. Ramos-Casals M, Solans R, Rosas J, et al. Primary Sjogren syndrome in Spain: clinical and immunologic expression in 1010 patients. Medicine (Baltimore) 2008;87:210–9.

114. Uffmann M, Kiener HP, Bankier AA, et al. Lung manifestation in asymptomatic patients with primary Sjogren syndrome: assessment with high resolution CT and pulmonary function tests. J Thorac Imaging 2001;16:282–9.

115. Koyama M, Johkoh T, Honda O, et al. Pulmonary involvement in primary Sjogren's syndrome: spectrum of pulmonary abnormalities and computed tomography findings in 60 patients. J Thorac Imaging 2001;16:290–6.

116. Franquet T, Gimenez A, Monill JM, et al. Primary Sjogren's syndrome and associated lung disease: CT findings in 50 patients. AJR Am J Roentgenol 1997;169:655–8.

117. Lohrmann C, Uhl M, Warnatz K, et al. High-resolution CT imaging of the lung for patients with primary Sjogren's syndrome. Eur J Radiol 2004;52:137–43.

118. Parambil JG, Myers JL, Lindell RM, et al. Interstitial lung disease in primary Sjogren syndrome. Chest 2006;130:1489–95.

119. Ito I, Nagai S, Kitaichi M, et al. Pulmonary manifestations of primary Sjogren's syndrome: a clinical, radiologic, and pathologic study. Am J Respir Crit Care Med 2005;171:632–8.

120. Yamadori I, Fujita J, Bandoh S, et al. Nonspecific interstitial pneumonia as pulmonary involvement of primary Sjogren's syndrome. Rheumatol Int 2002;22:89–92.

121. Nicholson AG. Classification of idiopathic interstitial pneumonias: making sense of the alphabet soup. Histopathology 2002;41:381–91.

122. Kokosi M, Riemer EC, Highland KB. Pulmonary involvement in Sjogren syndrome. Clin Chest Med 2010;31:489–500.

123. Honda O, Johkoh T, Ichikado K, et al. Differential diagnosis of lymphocytic interstitial pneumonia and malignant lymphoma on high-resolution CT. Am J Roentgenol 1999;173:71–4.

124. Jeong YJ, Lee KS, Chung MP, et al. Amyloidosis and lymphoproliferative disease in Sjogren syndrome: thin-section computed tomography findings and histopathologic comparisons. J Comput Assist Tomogr 2004;28:776–81.

125. Desai SR, Nicholson AG, Stewart S, et al. Benign pulmonary lymphocytic infiltration and amyloidosis: computed tomographic and pathologic features in three cases. J Thorac Imaging 1997;12:215–20.

126. Baqir M, Kluka EM, Aubry MC, et al. Amyloid-associated cystic lung disease in primary Sjogren's syndrome. Respir Med 2013;107:616–21.

127. Swanton J, Isenberg D. Mixed connective tissue disease: still crazy after all these years. Rheum Dis Clin North Am 2005;31:421–36, v.

128. Lazaro MA, Maldonado Cocco JA, Catoggio LJ, et al. Clinical and serologic characteristics of patients with overlap syndrome: is mixed connective tissue disease a distinct clinical entity? Medicine (Baltimore) 1989;68:58–65.

129. Aringer M, Steiner G, Smolen JS. Does mixed connective tissue disease exist? Yes. Rheum Dis Clin North Am 2005;31:411–20, v.
130. Gunnarsson R, Aalokken TM, Molberg O, et al. Prevalence and severity of interstitial lung disease in mixed connective tissue disease: a nationwide, cross-sectional study. Ann Rheum Dis 2012;71:1966–72.
131. Bodolay E, Szekanecz Z, Dévényi K, et al. Evaluation of interstitial lung disease in mixed connective tissue disease (MCTD). Rheumatology 2005;44:656–61.
132. Kozuka T, Johkoh T, Honda O, et al. Pulmonary involvement in mixed connective tissue disease: high-resolution CT findings in 41 patients. J Thorac Imaging 2001;16:94–8.
133. Saito Y, Terada M, Takada T, et al. Pulmonary involvement in mixed connective tissue disease: comparison with other collagen vascular diseases using high resolution CT. J Comput Assist Tomogr 2002;26:349–57.
134. Suda T, Kaida Y, Nakamura Y, et al. Acute exacerbation of interstitial pneumonia associated with collagen vascular diseases. Respir Med 2009;103:846–53.
135. Parambil JG, Myers JL, Ryu JH. Diffuse alveolar damage: uncommon manifestation of pulmonary involvement in patients with connective tissue diseases. Chest 2006;130:553–8.
136. Tachikawa R, Tomii K, Ueda H, et al. Clinical features and outcome of acute exacerbation of interstitial pneumonia: collagen vascular diseases-related versus idiopathic. Respiration 2012;83:20–7.
137. Mochizuki T, Aotsuka S, Satoh T. Clinical and laboratory features of lupus patients with complicating pulmonary disease. Respir Med 1999;93:95–101.
138. Grigor R, Edmonds J, Lewkonia R, et al. Systemic lupus erythematosus. A prospective analysis. Ann Rheum Dis 1978;37:121–8.
139. Estes D, Christian CL. The natural history of systemic lupus erythematosus by prospective analysis. Medicine (Baltimore) 1971;50:85–95.
140. Matthay RA, Schwarz MI, Petty TL, et al. Pulmonary manifestations of systemic lupus erythematosus: review of twelve cases of acute lupus pneumonitis. Medicine (Baltimore) 1975;54:397–409.
141. Hozumi H, Nakamura Y, Johkoh T, et al. Acute exacerbation in rheumatoid arthritis-associated interstitial lung disease: a retrospective case control study. BMJ Open 2013;3:e003132.
142. Rossi SE, Erasmus JJ, McAdams HP, et al. Pulmonary drug toxicity: radiologic and pathologic manifestations. Radiographics 2000;20:1245–59.
143. Cannon GW. Methotrexate pulmonary toxicity. Rheum Dis Clin North Am 1997; 23:917–37.
144. Sakai T, Noma S, Kurihara Y, et al. Leflunamide-related lung injury in patients with rheumatoid arthritis: imaging features. Mod Rheumatol 2005;15:173–9.
145. Savage RL, Highton J, Boyd IW, et al. Pneumonitis associated with leflunomide: a profile of New Zealand and Australian reports. Intern Med J 2006;36:162–9.
146. Sathi N, Chikura B, Kaushik VV, et al. How common is methotrexate pneumonitis? A large prospective study investigates. Clin Rheumatol 2012;31:79–83.
147. Carette S, Macher AM, Nussbaum A, et al. Severe, acute pulmonary disease in patients with systemic lupus erythematosus: ten years of experience at the National Institutes of Health. Semin Arthritis Rheum 1984;14:52–9.
148. Zamora MR, Warner ML, Tuder R, et al. Diffuse alveolar hemorrhage and systemic lupus erythematosus: clinical presentation, histology, survival, and outcome. Medicine 1997;76:192–202.
149. Schwab EP, Schumacher HR Jr, Freundlich B, et al. Pulmonary alveolar hemorrhage in systemic lupus erythematosus. Semin Arthritis Rheum 1993;23:8–15.

150. Santos-Ocampo AS, Mandell BF, Fessler BJ. Alveolar hemorrhage in systemic lupus erythematosus: presentation and management. Chest 2000;118:1083–90.
151. Cheah FK, Sheppard MN, Hansell DM. Computed tomography of diffuse pulmonary haemorrhage with pathological correlation. Clin Radiol 1993;48:89–93.
152. Murayama S, Murakami J, Yabuuchi H, et al. "Crazy paving appearance" on high resolution CT in various diseases. J Comput Assist Tomogr 1999;23:749–52.
153. Tyndall AJ, Bannert B, Vonk M, et al. Causes and risk factors for death in systemic sclerosis: a study from the EULAR Scleroderma Trials and Research (EUSTAR) database. Ann Rheum Dis 2010;69:1809–15.
154. Wallis RS, Broder MS, Wong JY, et al. Granulomatous infectious diseases associated with tumor necrosis factor antagonists. Clin Infect Dis 2004;38:1261–5.
155. Thavarajah K, Wu P, Rhew EJ, et al. Pulmonary complications of tumor necrosis factor-targeted therapy. Respir Med 2009;103:661–9.
156. Hagiwara K, Sato T, Takagi-Kobayashi S, et al. Acute exacerbation of preexisting interstitial lung disease after administration of etanercept for rheumatoid arthritis. J Rheumatol 2007;34:1151–4.
157. Pareja JG, Garland R, Koziel H. Use of adjunctive corticosteroids in severe adult non-HIV *Pneumocystis carinii* pneumonia. Chest 1998;113:1215–24.
158. Park IN, Kim DS, Shim TS, et al. Acute exacerbation of interstitial pneumonia other than idiopathic pulmonary fibrosis. Chest 2007;132:214–20.
159. Desai SR, Wells AU, Suntharalingam G, et al. Acute respiratory distress syndrome caused by pulmonary and extrapulmonary injury: a comparative CT study. Radiology 2001;218:689–93.
160. Owens CM, Evans TW, Keogh BF, et al. Computed tomography in established adult respiratory distress syndrome. Correlation with lung injury score. Chest 1994;106:1815–21.
161. Goodman LR, Fumagalli R, Tagliabue P, et al. Adult respiratory distress syndrome due to pulmonary and extrapulmonary causes: CT, clinical, and functional correlations. Radiology 1999;213:545–52.
162. Chung JH, Kradin RL, Greene RE, et al. CT predictors of mortality in pathology confirmed ARDS. Eur Radiol 2011;21:730–7.
163. Silver SF, Muller NL, Miller RR, et al. Hypersensitivity pneumonitis: evaluation with CT. Radiology 1989;173:441–5.
164. Lacasse Y, Selman M, Costabel U, et al. Clinical diagnosis of hypersensitivity pneumonitis. Am J Respir Crit Care Med 2003;168:952–8.
165. Hoeper MM. Pulmonary hypertension in collagen vascular disease. Eur Respir J 2002;19:571–6.
166. McLaughlin V, Humbert M, Coghlan G, et al. Pulmonary arterial hypertension: the most devastating vascular complication of systemic sclerosis. Rheumatology 2009;48:iii25–31.
167. Wells AU, Steen V, Valentini G. Pulmonary complications: one of the most challenging complications of systemic sclerosis. Rheumatology 2009;48:iii40–4.
168. Solomon JJ, Olson AL, Fischer A, et al. Scleroderma lung disease. Eur Respir Rev 2013;22:6–19.
169. Prakash UB. Respiratory complications in mixed connective tissue disease. Clin Chest Med 1998;19:733–46, ix.
170. Prabu A, Patel K, Yee CS, et al. Prevalence and risk factors for pulmonary arterial hypertension in patients with lupus. Rheumatology 2009;48:1506–11.
171. Kawut SM, Taichman DB, Archer-Chicko CL, et al. Haemodynamics and survival in patients with pulmonary artery hypertension related to systemic sclerosis. Chest 2003;123:344–50.

172. Kuriyama K, Gamsu G, Stern RG, et al. CT-determined pulmonary artery diameters in predicting pulmonary hypertension. Invest Radiol 1984;19: 16–22.

173. Ng CS, Wells AU, Padley SP. A CT sign of chronic pulmonary arterial hypertension: the ratio of main pulmonary artery to aortic diameter. J Thorac Imaging 1999;14:270–8.

174. Devaraj A, Wells AU, Meister MG, et al. The effect of diffuse pulmonary fibrosis on the reliability of CT signs of pulmonary hypertension. Radiology 2008;249: 1042–9.

175. Nolan RL, McAdams HP, Sporn TA, et al. Pulmonary cholesterol granulomas in patients with pulmonary artery hypertension: chest radiographic and CT findings. AJR Am J Roentgenol 1999;172:1317–9.

176. Luo YF, Robbins IM, Karatas M, et al. Frequency of pleural effusions in patients with pulmonary arterial hypertension associated with connective tissue diseases. Chest 2011;140:42–7.

177. Hill C, Nguyen A, Roder D, et al. Risk of cancer in patients with scleroderma: a population based cohort study. Ann Rheum Dis 2003;62:728–31.

178. Huang YL, Chen YJ, Lin MW, et al. Malignancies associated with dermatomyositis and polymyositis in Taiwan: a nationwide population-based study. Br J Dermatol 2009;161:854–60.

179. Bernatsky S, Boivin JF, Joseph L, et al. An international cohort study of cancer in systemic lupus erythematosus. Arthritis Rheum 2005;52:1481–90.

180. Rosenthal AK, McLaughlin JK, Gridley G, et al. Incidence of cancer among patients with systemic sclerosis. Cancer 1995;76:910–4.

181. Bin J, Bernatsky S, Gordon C, et al. Lung cancer in systemic lupus erythematosus. Lung Cancer 2007;56:303–6.

182. Hesselstrand R, Scheja A, Åkesson A. Mortality and causes of death in a Swedish series of systemic sclerosis patients. Ann Rheum Dis 1998;57:682–6.

183. Kassan SS, Thomas TL, Moutsopoulos HM, et al. Increased risk of lymphoma in sicca syndrome. Ann Intern Med 1978;89:888–92.

184. Buchbinder R, Hill CL. Malignancy in patients with inflammatory myopathy. Curr Rheumatol Rep 2002;4:415–26.

185. Moore OA, Goh N, Corte T, et al. Extent of disease on high-resolution computed tomography lung is a predictor of decline and mortality in systemic sclerosis-related interstitial lung disease. Rheumatology 2013;52:155–60.

186. Dawson JK, Fewins HE, Desmond J, et al. Predictors of progression of HRCT diagnosed fibrosing alveolitis in patients with rheumatoid arthritis. Ann Rheum Dis 2002;61:517–21.

187. Roth MD, Tseng CH, Clements PJ, et al. Predicting treatment outcomes and responder subsets in scleroderma-related interstitial lung disease. Arthritis Rheum 2011;63:2797–808.

188. Goh NS, Desai SR, Veeraraghavan S, et al. Interstitial lung disease in systemic sclerosis: a simple staging system. Am J Respir Crit Care Med 2008;177: 1248–54.

189. Edey AJ, Devaraj AA, Barker RP, et al. Fibrotic idiopathic interstitial pneumonias: HRCT findings that predict mortality. Eur Radiol 2011;21:1586–93.

190. Strange C, Highland KB. Interstitial lung disease in the patient who has connective tissue disease. Clin Chest Med 2004;25:549–59, vii.

191. Mosca M, Neri R, Bombardieri S. Undifferentiated connective tissue diseases (UCTD): a review of the literature and a proposal for preliminary classification criteria. Clin Exp Rheumatol 1999;17:615–20.

192. Homma Y, Ohtsuka Y, Tanimura K, et al. Can interstitial pneumonia as the sole presentation of collagen vascular diseases be differentiated from idiopathic interstitial pneumonia? Respiration 1995;62:248–51.
193. Tzelepis GE, Toya SP, Moutsopoulos HM. Occult connective tissue diseases mimicking idiopathic interstitial pneumonias. Eur Respir J 2008;31:11–20.
194. Fischer A, West SG, Swigris JJ, et al. Connective tissue disease-associated interstitial lung disease: a call for clarification. Chest 2010;138:251–6.

# Histopathology of Lung Disease in the Connective Tissue Diseases

Marina Vivero, MD, Robert F. Padera, MD, PhD*

## KEYWORDS

- Pathology • Histopathology • Interstitial lung disease • Connective tissue disease
- Rheumatoid arthritis • Scleroderma • Myositis

## KEY POINTS

- Although there is substantial histologic overlap among the pulmonary manifestations of different connective tissue diseases (CTDs), certain patterns may favor 1 CTD over another; occasionally, distinctive histologic clues may be present.
- CTDs may present with acute, subacute, and/or chronic pleuropulmonary manifestations, often mixed within the same biopsy, representing ongoing disease.
- Patients with CTD may be taking immunosuppressive medications and are vulnerable to certain infections; both of these can result in histologic changes that are similar to direct pulmonary manifestations of the underlying CTD and can represent diagnostic dilemmas for the pathologist.
- A multidisciplinary approach involving the pathologist, rheumatologist, pulmonologist, and radiologist allows for correlation of the clinical, radiologic, and pathologic findings to arrive at the proper diagnosis.

## INTRODUCTION

The pathologic correlates of interstitial lung disease (ILD) secondary to connective tissue disease (CTD) comprise a diverse group of histologic patterns that can vary greatly within a given CTD and may in fact display significant overlap between distinct CTDs.[1] Lung biopsies in patients with CTD-associated ILD tend to demonstrate simultaneous involvement of multiple anatomic compartments of the lung, including the airways, alveolar septa, alveolar spaces, pleura, and vasculature, and often demonstrate acute, subacute, and chronic lesions within the same specimen, indicating an ongoing pathophysiologic process.[1,2] All CTDs can result in nonspecific histologic

The authors have no disclosures to make.
Department of Pathology, Brigham and Women's Hospital, 75 Francis Street, Boston, MA 02115, USA
* Corresponding author.
*E-mail address:* rpadera@partners.org

patterns that are essentially indistinguishable from the idiopathic interstitial pneumonias; however, in the setting of known CTD, the probability that the lung findings are caused by the patient's underlying systemic disease must be considered.[3,4] Certain histologic patterns do tend to predominate in each defined CTD, and it is possible in many cases to confirm connective tissue-associated lung disease and guide patient management using surgical lung biopsy.

Some pulmonary pathologies seen in patients with CTD may not be a direct manifestation of the effect of CTD on the lung, but may be related to therapy or to other systemic complications of the patient's CTD. These conditions can result in significant histologic changes that can make it difficult to determine which findings can be truly be ascribed to involvement by the patient's CTD.[5–7] For example, a patient with rheumatoid arthritis (RA) treated with methotrexate may develop a cellular nonspecific interstitial pneumonitis (NSIP) secondary to drug toxicity; this may mimic cellular NSIP that could represent the bona fide onset of RA-associated ILD, or it could mimic the histologic pattern of a viral pneumonia to which the patient would be predisposed secondary to immunosuppression. The recognition and contextualization of these processes are best accomplished via review by a multidisciplinary team, including pathologists with specialized training in thoracic pathology or significant experience reading nonneoplastic surgical lung biopsies, rheumatologists, pulmonologists, and radiologists. This article will cover the pulmonary pathologies seen in RA, systemic sclerosis, myositis, systemic lupus erythematosus, Sjögren syndrome, and mixed CTD.

## HISTOLOGY OF LUNG DISEASE IN RHEUMATOID ARTHRITIS

Perhaps more so than any of the other CTDs, lung disease in patients with RA exhibits a wide variety of histopathologic patterns that can affect all of the major compartments of the lung. Pleural effusion and pleuritis are common initial pleuropulmonary manifestations of RA and may be appreciated grossly and microscopically as acute fibrinous pleuritis, fibrous pleural thickening, and/or pleural adhesions.[8–10] Cytologic preparations of pleural fluid may have characteristic aggregates of amorphous debris and degenerated neutrophils.[11] Single or multiple rheumatoid nodules (**Fig. 1**) may be

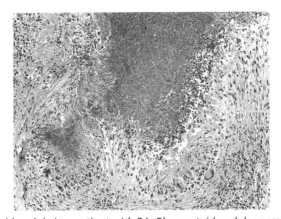

**Fig. 1.** Rheumatoid nodule in a patient with RA. Rheumatoid nodules possess a central area of amorphous, eosinophilic necrobiosis surrounded by a rim of epithelioid histiocytes and occasional giant cells. A mixed inflammatory infiltrate including occasional neutrophils may line the inner perimeter of the histiocyte rim, and there may be finely granular basophilic material within areas of necrobiosis, imparting a dirty appearance at low power. 100 × original magnification.

found in the pleura, interlobular septa, or alveolar interstitium; although not the most common manifestation, they are considered the most specific finding of RA-ILD. These nodules, which can measure up to 2 to 3 cm, are identical to those seen in the subcutaneous tissues, consisting of sterile central necrobiosis surrounded by epithelioid histiocytes.[5,8,9]

The most frequent histologic patterns of ILD among RA patients are NSIP (**Fig. 2**), followed closely by usual interstitial pneumonia (UIP) (**Figs. 3** and **4**), accounting for 30% to 67% and 13% to 57% of RA-associated ILD, respectively.[2,3,12–17] Some studies have noted an equal or greater incidence of UIP histology in RA-ILD, although smaller sample sizes and the high frequency of both ILD patterns among this patient population may account for the discrepancy.[14,18] The histologic appearance of RA-associated NSIP (RA-NSIP) or UIP (RA-UIP) is identical to that seen in idiopathic NSIP and UIP, although the occurrence of more prominent interstitial lymphoid aggregates, either within alveolar septal walls or associated with small airways, has been noted in several studies.[5,9] Indeed, the presence of lymphoid aggregates, and specifically germinal centers, has been reported to be significantly greater in RA-UIP than in UIP, and has been suggested to be a distinguishing feature of RA-ILD.[12,15,16,19] Similarly, the frequency of fibroblast foci has been reported to be lesser in RA-UIP than in idiopathic UIP.[3,16]

Various types of inflammatory airway disease including bronchiectasis, chronic bronchitis, and follicular bronchiolitis are often seen as a secondary finding in a background of NSIP or UIP.[17,20,21] Acute and subacute processes such as diffuse alveolar damage (DAD) and organizing pneumonia (OP) can be seen in patients with established RA-ILD, often in the clinical setting of an acute exacerbation, but they can occasionally represent the initial pulmonary manifestation of RA.[5,14,18,22] Vasculitis, capillaritis, and pulmonary hemorrhage are rare acute manifestations of RA-ILD; chronic vascular manifestations, when present, are usually a result of underlying fibrotic lung disease.[23]

## HISTOLOGY OF LUNG DISEASE IN SYSTEMIC SCLEROSIS (SCLERODERMA)

ILD occurs in up to 80% of patients with systemic sclerosis (SSc), making ILD more prevalent in SSc than in any other CTD. The most characteristic histologic features

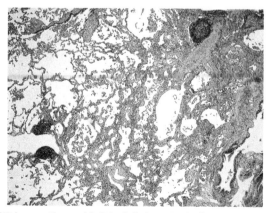

**Fig. 2.** Cellular NSIP in a patient with RA. Cellular NSIP is characterized by uniform expansion of the alveolar septal interstitium by a chronic inflammatory infiltrate composed primarily of small lymphocytes intermixed with occasional plasma cells and histiocytes. Prominent lymphoid aggregates and germinal centers are characteristic of RA. 20 × original magnification.

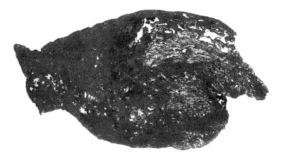

**Fig. 3.** UIP in a patient with RA. The UIP pattern is characterized by patchy, predominantly subpleural interstitial fibrosis. Interstitial fibrosis in UIP, unlike NSIP, appears temporally heterogenous, with some areas of dense eosinophilic or elastotic mature interstitial collagen and other areas of looser, immature myxoid collagenous matrix with discrete, lens-shaped nodes of fibroblastic proliferation (fibroblast foci). These areas of involvement often demonstrate a characteristic, sharply demarcated interface with completely uninvolved lung parenchyma. As in RA-NSIP, an increased number of lymphoid aggregates and germinal centers are present in RA-UIP. 1 × original magnification.

of ILD in SSc are dense interstitial fibrosis and pulmonary hypertensive vascular changes.[24,25] The most common pattern of interstitial fibrosis in SSc is fibrotic NSIP (**Fig. 5**), manifesting as dense, paucicellular interstitial fibrosis that maintains the underlying lung architecture and often spares the immediate subpleural area.[26–28] As the lung disease progresses, the areas of fibrosis may become confluent and appear as honeycomb or end-stage lung. Patients with SSc may also manifest their ILD as a typical UIP pattern with temporal and spatial heterogeneity, in contrast to the diffusely uniform fibrosis of NSIP. The pulmonary hypertensive vascular changes (**Fig. 6**) are manifested as concentric intimal thickening by fibromyxoid tissue and mild medial hypertrophy leading to thickened and stenotic pulmonary arterioles. The degree of pulmonary hypertensive changes is often more severe and out of proportion to the degree of interstitial fibrosis.[29] Although true vasculitis and pulmonary hemorrhage can occasionally be seen, it is a fairly uncommon feature in this disease.[30] Patients with SSc often have esophageal dysmotility with associated gastrointestinal reflux; this can

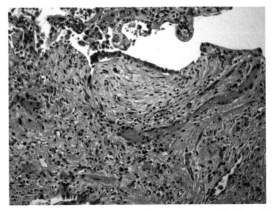

**Fig. 4.** UIP in a patient with RA. A fibroblastic focus is seen at the interface between dense fibrosis and normal lung. 100 × original magnification.

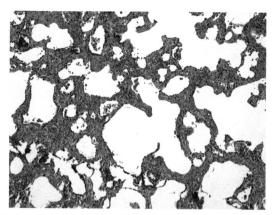

**Fig. 5.** Fibrotic NSIP in a patient with SSc. Fibrotic NSIP is characterized by dense, paucicellular interstitial fibrosis that largely maintains the underlying lung architecture and is spatially and temporally homogeneous. 40 × original magnification.

lead to superimposed aspiration pneumonia that may or may not be clinically apparent but can complicate the interpretation of the surgical lung biopsy.

## HISTOLOGY OF LUNG DISEASE IN MYOSITIS

Chronic pulmonary disease in polymyositis and dermatomyositis (PM-DM) consists of varying degrees of cellular interstitial pneumonitis that are best characterized as NSIP (**Fig. 7**).[2,6,22,31–35] Most case series have described varying degrees of fibrosis accompanying the cellular interstitial infiltrates of PM-DM, including 1 study indicating approximately a 40% prevalence of cellular NSIP and 53% prevalence of mixed cellular and fibrotic NSIP in myositis patients, with only rare cases of pure fibrotic NSIP.[33] The OP pattern (**Fig. 8**) can be seen in PM-DM patients, either as an isolated manifestation or superimposed on a background of NSIP, and it has been histologically confirmed to resolve with steroid treatment.[32,34,36] UIP pattern histology has been

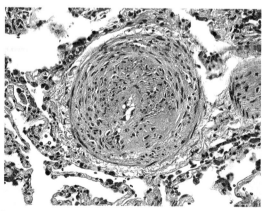

**Fig. 6.** Pulmonary hypertensive vascular disease in a patient with SSc. The arteriolar wall is thickened and the lumen narrowed by a fibrointimal proliferation with no significant inflammation. 200 × original magnification.

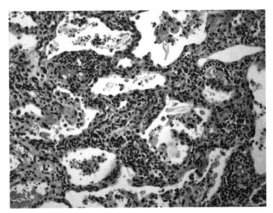

**Fig. 7.** Cellular NSIP in a patient with PM. There is a dense lymphocytic infiltrate that expands the alveolar walls but does not distort the underlying lung architecture. In this case, intra-alveolar macrophages are abundant as well. 100 × original magnification.

described in PM-DM and, similar to RA-UIP, it often contains at least moderately cellular areas consisting of lymphoplasmacytic or mononuclear infiltrates.[2,16,31,34,36] The UIP pattern may arise more frequently in patients with the antisynthetase antibody Jo-1. DAD is occasionally seen as a more acute manifestation of PM-DM lung disease in the clinical setting of acute exacerbation of underlying chronic lung disease, and it typically carries a poor prognosis similar to DAD associated with the clinical entity of acute respiratory distress syndrome.[22,33,36,37] Other more florid cellular manifestations of ILD, such as follicular bronchiolitis and lymphoid interstitial pneumonia (LIP) are rare in PM-DM.[1,7,34] Other rare manifestations of ILD associated with PM-DM include diffuse alveolar hemorrhage (DAH), pleuritis, airway involvement, and vasculitis.[1,38]

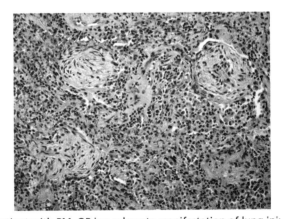

**Fig. 8.** OP in a patient with PM. OP is a subacute manifestation of lung injury that has been described as a manifestation of all connective tissue diseases. Histologically, OP has been characterized by rounded to elongated plugs of fibroblasts embedded in a blue-tinted immature collagenous matrix within alveolar spaces, alveolar ducts, and occasionally the terminal airways. An associated interstitial lymphocytic infiltrate often accompanies the fibroblastic proliferation and may be brisk. 100 × original magnification.

## HISTOLOGY OF LUNG DISEASE IN SYSTEMIC LUPUS ERYTHEMATOSUS

Pleuritis is the most frequent pleuropulmonary manifestation of systemic lupus erythematosus (SLE), and it appears histologically as nonspecific inflammation, fibrin deposition, and pleural fibrosis (**Fig. 9**).[39–43] Cytologic preparations of pleural fluid from SLE patients may show pathognomonic lupus erythematosis cells consisting of neutrophils or macrophages with intracytoplasmic remnants of degenerated nuclei.

Pulmonary involvement in SLE is usually acute in nature and presents clinically as acute lupus pneumonitis (ALP), which correlates to a variety of nonspecific acute and organizing lung injury patterns (**Fig. 10**) in surgical lung biopsies.[44] Acute and organizing diffuse alveolar damage, with fibrin microthrombi, hemorrhage, and hyaline membranes in various stages of fibroblastic organization, is the most frequently reported manifestation of lupus lung disease.[43,45–47] OP also seems to be a common finding among studies of lupus pneumonitis.[48–50] Finally, DAH is a potentially fatal acute complication of SLE, possibly as a result of capillary immune complex deposition, and can be seen as fresh hemorrhage or aggregates of hemosiderin laden (**Fig. 11**) within alveolar spaces and alveolar septa, with or without capillaritis.[39–41,43,51–53]

Chronic lung disease is also seen in patients with SLE. Most studies describe mononuclear or lymphoplasmacytic interstitial and peribronchiolar infiltrates of variable intensity in a cellular NSIP pattern with lesser degrees of fibrosis.[1,40,42,48,53,54] Pulmonary vascular disease leading to pulmonary hypertension can occur in SLE, possibly secondary to chronic thromboembolic disease or repeated episodes of vasculitis with healing. The morphology of the vascular disease can range from active vasculitis to chronic intimal thickening to plexiform lesions. Other patterns of chronic lung disease such as UIP, diffuse interstitial fibrosis, LIP, and amyloidosis have been reported, but these are rare.[2,39,40,48,50,52–54]

## HISTOLOGY OF LUNG DISEASE IN SJÖGREN SYNDROME

Sjögren syndrome (SjS)-associated ILD (SjS-ILD) presents with a spectrum of cellular chronic interstitial pneumonia and airway disease that ranges from a minimally cellular NSIP pattern to more florid patterns of lymphoplasmacytic infiltration such as follicular

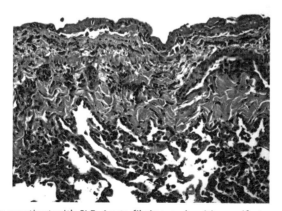

**Fig. 9.** Pleuritis in a patient with SLE. Acute fibrinous pleuritis manifests as a layer of hypereosinophilic fibrin on the pleural surface, usually with chronic inflammation in the visceral pleura underneath. Over time, the pleura may become fibrotic with diminished active inflammation. 100 × original magnification.

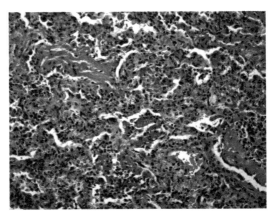

**Fig. 10.** ALP in a patient with SLE. The histology of ALP involves a lung injury pattern with diffuse interstitial inflammation, reactive pneumocyte hyperplasia, and alveolar fibrin present either as hyaline membranes or as acute fibrinous pneumonia. There may be variable degrees of organization of this process depending on when the biopsy was performed relative to the onset of symptoms. 100 × original magnification.

bronchiolitis, lymphoid interstitial hyperplasia, and LIP. NSIP as a cellular, fibrotic, or mixed pattern is the more commonly reported histologic pattern of SjS-ILD in recent studies.[22,55,56] LIP (**Fig. 12**) lies on the other end of the spectrum of cellular chronic interstitial pneumonitis seen in SjS-ILD and is characterized by a florid peribronchiolar and interstitial lymphoplasmacytic infiltrate that significantly expands the alveolar septa, is usually associated with germinal centers, and may occasionally contain rare poorly formed non-necrotizing granulomas. Among the CTDs, LIP is most often associated with SjS and may represent a precursor lesion that is associated with

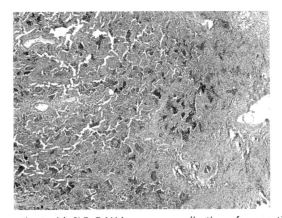

**Fig. 11.** DAH in a patient with SLE. DAH is a rare complication of connective tissue disease and is most commonly seen in SLE. The predominant histologic findings in DAH are numerous intra-alveolar and interstitial aggregates of hemosiderin-laden macrophages (as seen in the image), with or without evidence of fresh hemorrhage. Capillaritis may be an associated finding in DAH, but may be subtle or entirely absent, and is characterized by neutrophilic alveolar septal infiltrates accompanied by fibrinoid necrosis and basophilic neutrophil nuclear dust. 10 × original magnification.

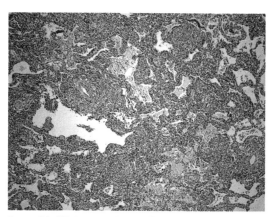

**Fig. 12.** LIP in a patient with SjS. LIP constitutes the extreme end of the spectrum of chronic cellular interstitial pneumonitis that can be seen in SjS and is characterized by florid airway-centered and alveolar interstitial chronic inflammatory infiltrates. Germinal centers and occasional poorly formed non-necrotizing granulomas or histiocytic aggregates can be seen. Destructive or aggressively infiltrative lymphoid populations are not typical of LIP and should raise the possibility of lymphoma. 20 × original magnification.

the significantly higher incidence of lymphoma in SjS patients.[22,56–59] Although the prevalence of LIP in SjS patients is estimated to be 0.9%, approximately 25% of patients with LIP histology are thought to have SjS.[59]

Involvement of the large and small airways in SjS is common. Airway involvement is thought to be analogous to the inflammatory findings in the salivary glands and upper respiratory tract, and it manifests as lymphoplasmacytic infiltrates of varying intensity ranging from mild chronic bronchiolitis to follicular bronchiolitis, which is characterized by nodular lymphocytic infiltrates with reactive germinal centers in an exquisitely bronchiolocentric distribution (**Fig. 13**).[56,59,60]

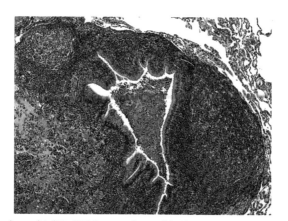

**Fig. 13.** Follicular bronchiolitis (FB) in a patient with SjS. FB is most commonly seen in connective tissue associated lung disease as part of the spectrum of chronic cellular interstitial pneumonitis that typifies SjS. Histologically, FB consists of a bronchiolocentric proliferation of lymphoid tissue with occasional germinal centers. The lymphoid infiltrates may or may not extend into the alveolar septal interstitium immediately surrounding the small airways. 20 × original magnification.

Other histologic patterns of interstitial lung disease, such as UIP, DAD, OP, and pleuritis, are much less common in patients with SjS. The acute and subacute patterns are most often superimposed on a background of chronic ILD in the setting of an acute exacerbation.

## HISTOLOGY OF LUNG DISEASE IN MIXED CONNECTIVE TISSUE DISEASE

Patients who have anti-(U1)snRNP antibodies manifesting some features of DM, PM, SLE, or SSc (but not meeting formal diagnostic criteria) are labeled as having mixed CTD (MCTD). Many of these patients will develop additional clinical and laboratory findings and eventually declare themselves as having one of the specific CTDs. Consistent with the clinical phenotype, the pulmonary manifestations of MCTD in any given patient may reflect any of the patterns discussed previously for the specific CTDs.

Acute fibrinous and chronic organizing pleuritis with pleural adhesions is a common finding in MCTD and appears similar to pleural disease related to other causes.[61] Organizing pneumonia and diffuse alveolar damage have been occasionally described in MCTD patients and have been suggested to represent acute exacerbations of underlying pulmonary disease.[49,62] Although pulmonary fibrosis with radiologic features of both NSIP and UIP has been described, histologic descriptions of chronic ILD in MCTD are scarce, limited to case reports or small series, and usually lack definitive histologic classification.[62–64]

Pulmonary vascular disease is a prominent and often predominant feature of MCTD-associated lung involvement, correlating with the clinical manifestations of severe and sometimes fatal pulmonary hypertension. The histologic changes include medial muscular hypertrophy, intimal fibromyxoid hyperplasia, and endothelial hyperplasia.[63,65] Plexiform arteriopathy can occasionally be seen in advanced cases. The sequelae of thromboembolic disease in the form of eccentric intimal proliferation have been reported in lung biopsies of patients with MCTD as a manifestation of CTD-associated hypercoagulability.[61] These vascular findings can be seen as an isolated finding or with concomitant interstitial fibrosis; however, when fibrosis is present, it is usually not extensive enough to explain the degree of vasculopathy, and the vascular findings are therefore considered to be a separate primary process.[65]

## HISTOLOGIC DIFFERENTIAL DIAGNOSIS OF LUNG DISEASE IN CONNECTIVE TISSUE DISEASES

The histologic differential diagnosis in cases of suspected pulmonary involvement by CTD can be broad and is compounded by the significant histologic overlap among pulmonary manifestations of CTD, by the immunosuppressed nature of the patients, and by various treatments that may induce histologic changes in the lung.[5,66] Each of the patterns of lung disease (ie, UIP, NSIP, OP, LIP) mentioned previously carries its own differential diagnosis that includes pulmonary involvement by one or more of the CTDs. There are several nonconnective tissue etiologies that cut across many of these patterns that should be considered. Various infections can mimic many of these patterns: viral infection can produce a cellular NSIP pattern, resolving bacterial pneumonia can produce an OP pattern, and invasive fungal or mycobacterial infection can produce necrotizing granulomas resembling those seen in granulomatosis with polyangiitis.[67] Pulmonary toxicity from certain medications can produce many of these injury patterns, particularly OP, cellular NSIP, and DAD. Many therapies for CTD including immunosuppressive agents such as methotrexate, cyclophosphamide, and possibly tumor necrosis factor (TNF)-α inhibitors can give rise to pulmonary pathologies and can present years after the offending drug has been discontinued.[4,66,68] Vasculitis and lupus-like syndromes are also potential pulmonary complications of immunosuppressive drugs.[66] Pulmonary injury caused by inhaled or aspirated material, either from one or multiple exposures, can lead to bronchiolitis and bronchiectasis that can enter into the differential of UIP, OP, DAD, or DAH. Chronic hypersensitivity pneumonitis is in the differential diagnosis of UIP and NSIP. Lymphoproliferative disorders, which can arise in the setting of certain CTDs such as SjS, can mimic cellular NSIP and LIP histologically, radiologically, and clinically, and need to be ruled out when the inflammatory infiltrate is unusually florid.[22,55,69–72] Of course, most of the histologic patterns, particularly UIP, have idiopathic forms that occur in the absence of CTD. On the other hand, it is also the case that any of these patterns can be the initial manifestation of a patient's yet to be clinically diagnosed CTD.[19]

## SUMMARY

ILD is common in patients with CTDs. Many of the histologic patterns of the idiopathic interstitial pneumonidites such as UIP, cellular and/or fibrotic NSIP, LIP, DAD, and OP can also be seen in patients with CTD; occasionally, the pulmonary manifestations of CTD may precede formal diagnosis of the underlying CTD. The pulmonary manifestations of CTD can result from the direct involvement of the CTD on the lung, from drug reactions from the patient's medications, or from infections to which the patient is predisposed from his or her autoimmune disease and treatment thereof. The histologic changes seen in a given patient's surgical lung biopsy may result from any or all of these, and correlation with the clinical scenario is critical in arriving at the proper diagnosis.

## REFERENCES

1. Schneider F, Gruden J, Tazelaar HD, et al. Pleuropulmonary pathology in patients with rheumatic disease. Arch Pathol Lab Med 2012;136:1242–52.
2. Tansey D, Wells AU, Colby TV, et al. Variations in histological patterns of interstitial pneumonia between connective tissue disorders and their relationship to prognosis. Histopathology 2004;44:585–96.
3. Cipriani NA, Strek M, Noth I, et al. Pathologic quantification of connective tissue disease-associated versus idiopathic usual interstitial pneumonia. Arch Pathol Lab Med 2012;136:1253–8.
4. Travis WD, Costabel U, Hansell DM, et al. An official American Thoracic Society/European Respiratory Society statement: update of the international multidisciplinary classification of the idiopathic interstitial pneumonias. Am J Respir Crit Care Med 2013;188:733–48.
5. Yousem SA, Colby TV, Carrington CB. Lung biopsy in rheumatoid arthritis. Am Rev Respir Dis 1985;131:770–7.
6. Fathi M, Lundberg IE. Interstitial lung disease in polymyositis and dermatomyositis. Curr Opin Rheumatol 2005;17:701–6.
7. Kalluri M, Oddis CV. Pulmonary manifestations of the idiopathic inflammatory myopathies. Clin Chest Med 2010;31:501–12.
8. Macfarlane JD, Dieppe PA, Rigden BG, et al. Pulmonary and pleural lesions in rheumatoid disease. Br J Dis Chest 1978;72:288–300.
9. Hakala M, Pääkkö P, Huhti E, et al. Open lung biopsy of patients with rheumatoid arthritis. Clin Rheumatol 1990;9:452–60.
10. Hashimoto K, Nakanishi H, Yamasaki A, et al. Pulmonary findings without the influence of therapy in a patient with rheumatoid arthritis: an autopsy case. J Med Invest 2007;54:340–4.

11. De las Casas LE, Morales AM, Boman DA, et al. Laparoscopic aspiration cytology in rheumatoid ascites: a case report. Acta Cytol 2010;54:1123–6.
12. Turesson C, Matteson EL, Colby TV, et al. Increased CD4+ T cell infiltrates in rheumatoid arthritis-associated interstitial pneumonitis compared with idiopathic interstitial pneumonitis. Arthritis Rheum 2005;52:73–9.
13. Lee HK, Kim DS, Yoo B, et al. Histopathologic pattern and clinical features of rheumatoid arthritis-associated interstitial lung disease. Chest 2005;127:2019–27.
14. Yoshinouchi T, Ohtsuki Y, Fujita J, et al. Nonspecific interstitial pneumonia pattern as pulmonary involvement of rheumatoid arthritis. Rheumatol Int 2005;26:121–5.
15. Atkins SR, Turesson C, Myers JL, et al. Morphologic and quantitative assessment of CD20+ B cell infiltrates in rheumatoid arthritis-associated nonspecific interstitial pneumonia and usual interstitial pneumonia. Arthritis Rheum 2006;54:635–41.
16. Song JW, Do KH, Kim MY, et al. Pathologic and radiologic differences between idiopathic and collagen vascular disease-related usual interstitial pneumonia. Chest 2009;136:23–30.
17. Nakamura Y, Suda T, Kaida Y, et al. Rheumatoid lung disease: prognostic analysis of 54 biopsy-proven cases. Respir Med 2012;106:1164–9.
18. Hozumi H, Nakamura Y, Johkoh T, et al. Acute exacerbation in rheumatoid arthritis-associated interstitial lung disease: a retrospective case control study. BMJ Open 2013;3:e003132.
19. Kono M, Nakamura Y, Enomoto N, et al. Usual interstitial pneumonia preceding collagen vascular disease: a retrospective case control study of patients initially diagnosed with idiopathic pulmonary fibrosis. PLoS One 2014;9:e94775.
20. Yousem SA, Colby TV, Carrington CB. Follicular bronchitis/bronchiolitis. Hum Pathol 1985;16:700–6.
21. Devouassoux G, Cottin V, Lioté H, et al. Characterisation of severe obliterative bronchiolitis in rheumatoid arthritis. Eur Respir J 2009;33:1053–61.
22. Parambil JG, Myers JL, Lindell RM, et al. Interstitial lung disease in primary Sjögren syndrome. Chest 2006;130:1489–95.
23. Schwarz MI, Zamora MR, Hodges TN, et al. Isolated pulmonary capillaritis and diffuse alveolar hemorrhage in rheumatoid arthritis and mixed connective tissue disease. Chest 1998;113:1609–15.
24. Fischer A, Swigris JJ, Groshong SD, et al. Clinically significant interstitial lung disease in limited scleroderma: histopathology, clinical features and survival. Chest 2008;134:601–5.
25. Kim EA, Lee KS, Johkoh T, et al. Interstitial lung diseases associated with collagen vascular diseases: radiologic and histopathologic findings. Radiographics 2002;22:S151–65.
26. Bouros D, Wells AU, Nicholson AG, et al. Histopathologic subsets of fibrosing alveolitis in patients with systemic sclerosis and their relationship to outcome. Am J Respir Crit Care Med 2002;165:1581–6.
27. Parra ER, Otani LH, de Carvalho EF, et al. Systemic sclerosis and idiopathic interstitial pneumonia: histomorphometric differences in lung biopsies. J Bras Pneumol 2009;35:529–40.
28. Fujita J, Yoshinouchi T, Ohtsuki Y, et al. Non-specific interstitial pneumonia as pulmonary involvement of systemic sclerosis. Ann Rheum Dis 2001;60:281–3.
29. Yousem SA. The pulmonary pathologic manifestations of the CREST syndrome. Hum Pathol 1990;21:467–74.

30. Griffin MT, Robb JD, Martin JR. Diffuse alveolar haemorrhage associated with progressive systemic sclerosis. Thorax 1990;45:903–4.

31. Duncan PE, Griffin JP, Garcia A, et al. Fibrosing alveolitis in polymyositis. A review of histologically confirmed cases. Am J Med 1974;57:621–6.

32. Schwarz MI, Matthay RA, Sahn SA, et al. Interstitial lung disease in polymyositis and dermatomyositis: analysis of six cases and review of the literature. Medicine (Baltimore) 1976;55:89–104.

33. Douglas WW, Tazelaar HD, Hartman TE, et al. Polymyositis-dermatomyositis-associated interstitial lung disease. Am J Respir Crit Care Med 2001;164:1182–5.

34. Cottin V, Thivolet-Béjui F, Reynaud-Gaubert M, et al. Interstitial lung disease in amyopathic dermatomyositis, dermatomyositis and polymyositis. Eur Respir J 2003;22:245–50.

35. Koreeda Y, Higashimoto I, Yamamoto M, et al. Clinical and pathological findings of interstitial lung disease patients with anti-aminoacyl-tRNA synthetase autoantibodies. Intern Med 2010;49:361–9.

36. Tazelaar HD, Viggiano RW, Pickersgill J, et al. Interstitial lung disease in polymyositis and dermatomyositis. Clinical features and prognosis as correlated with histologic findings. Am Rev Respir Dis 1990;141:727–33.

37. Matsuki Y, Yamashita H, Takahashi Y, et al. Diffuse alveolar damage in patients with dermatomyositis: a six-case series. Mod Rheumatol 2012;22:243–8.

38. Schwarz MI, Sutarik JM, Nick JA, et al. Pulmonary capillaritis and diffuse alveolar hemorrhage. A primary manifestation of polymyositis. Am J Respir Crit Care Med 1995;151:2037–40.

39. Kinney WW, Angelillo VA. Bronchiolitis in systemic lupus erythematosus. Chest 1982;82:646–9.

40. Wiedemann HP, Matthay RA. Pulmonary manifestations of systemic lupus erythematosus. J Thorac Imaging 1992;7:1–18.

41. Zamora MR, Warner ML, Tuder R, et al. Diffuse alveolar hemorrhage and systemic lupus erythematosus. Clinical presentation, histology, survival, and outcome. Medicine (Baltimore) 1997;76:192–202.

42. Keane MP, Lynch JP. Pleuropulmonary manifestations of systemic lupus erythematosus. Thorax 2000;55:159–66.

43. Kim JS, Lee KS, Koh EM, et al. Thoracic involvement of systemic lupus erythematosus: clinical, pathologic, and radiologic findings. J Comput Assist Tomogr 2000;24:9–18.

44. Lamblin C, Bergoin C, Saelens T, et al. Interstitial lung diseases in collagen vascular diseases. Eur Respir J Suppl 2001;32:69s–80s.

45. Haupt HM, Moore GW, Hutchins GM. The lung in systemic lupus erythematosus. Analysis of the pathologic changes in 120 patients. Am J Med 1981;71:791–8.

46. Lynch JP, Hunninghake GW. Pulmonary complications of collagen vascular disease. Annu Rev Med 1992;43:17–35.

47. Cheema GS, Quismorio FP. Interstitial lung disease in systemic lupus erythematosus. Curr Opin Pulm Med 2000;6:424–9.

48. Matthay RA, Schwarz MI, Petty TL, et al. Pulmonary manifestations of systemic lupus erythematosus: review of twelve cases of acute lupus pneumonitis. Medicine (Baltimore) 1975;54:397–409.

49. Gammon RB, Bridges TA, al-Nezir H, et al. Bronchiolitis obliterans organizing pneumonia associated with systemic lupus erythematosus. Chest 1992;102:1171–4.

50. Gutsche M, Rosen GD, Swigris JJ. Connective tissue disease-associated interstitial lung disease: a review. Curr Respir Care Rep 2012;1:224–32.

51. Eagen JW, Memoli VA, Roberts JL, et al. Pulmonary hemorrhage in systemic lupus erythematosus. Medicine (Baltimore) 1978;57:545–60.
52. Pines A, Kaplinsky N, Olchovsky D, et al. Pleuro-pulmonary manifestations of systemic lupus erythematosus: clinical features of its subgroups. Prognostic and therapeutic implications. Chest 1985;88:129–35.
53. Weinrib L, Sharma OP, Quismorio FP. A long-term study of interstitial lung disease in systemic lupus erythematosus. Semin Arthritis Rheum 1990;20:48–56.
54. Eisenberg H, Dubois EL, Sherwin RP, et al. Diffuse interstitial lung disease in systemic lupus erythematosus. Ann Intern Med 1973;79:37–45.
55. Ito I, Nagai S, Kitaichi M, et al. Pulmonary manifestations of primary Sjögren's syndrome: a clinical, radiologic, and pathologic study. Am J Respir Crit Care Med 2005;171:632–8.
56. Shi JH, Liu HR, Xu WB, et al. Pulmonary manifestations of Sjögren's syndrome. Respiration 2009;78:377–86.
57. Strimlan CV, Rosenow EC, Divertie MB, et al. Pulmonary manifestations of Sjögren's syndrome. Chest 1976;70:354–61.
58. Dalvi V, Gonzalez EB, Lovett L. Lymphocytic interstitial pneumonitis (LIP) in Sjögren's syndrome: a case report and a review of the literature. Clin Rheumatol 2007; 26:1339–43.
59. Kokosi M, Riemer EC, Highland KB. Pulmonary involvement in Sjögren syndrome. Clin Chest Med 2010;31:489–500.
60. Papiris SA, Maniati M, Constantopoulos SH, et al. Lung involvement in primary Sjögren's syndrome is mainly related to the small airway disease. Ann Rheum Dis 1999;58:61–4.
61. Hant FN, Herpel LB, Silver RM. Pulmonary manifestations of scleroderma and mixed connective tissue disease. Clin Chest Med 2010;31:433–49.
62. Watanabe Y, Koyama S, Moriguchi M, et al. Rapidly progressive respiratory failure in mixed connective tissue disease: report of an autopsy case. Intern Med 2012;51:3415–9.
63. Bull TM, Fagan KA, Badesch DB. Pulmonary vascular manifestations of mixed connective tissue disease. Rheum Dis Clin North Am 2005;31:451–64.
64. Bryson T, Sundaram B, Khanna D, et al. Connective tissue disease-associated interstitial pneumonia and idiopathic interstitial pneumonia: similarity and difference. Semin Ultrasound CT MR 2014;35:29–38.
65. Sullivan WD, Hurst DJ, Harmon CE, et al. A prospective evaluation emphasizing pulmonary involvement in patients with mixed connective tissue disease. Medicine (Baltimore) 1984;63:92–107.
66. Perez-Alvarez R, Perez-de-Lis M, Diaz-Lagares C, et al. Interstitial lung disease induced or exacerbated by TNF-targeted therapies: analysis of 122 cases. Semin Arthritis Rheum 2011;41:256–64.
67. Aubry MC. Necrotizing granulomatous inflammation: what does it mean if your special stains are negative? Mod Pathol 2012;25:S31–8.
68. Myers JL, Limper AH, Swensen SJ. Drug-induced lung disease: a pragmatic classification incorporating HRCT appearances. Semin Respir Crit Care Med 2003;24:445–54.
69. Carrillo J, Restrepo CS, Rosado de Christenson M, et al. Lymphoproliferative lung disorders: a radiologic-pathologic overview. Part I: reactive disorders. Semin Ultrasound CT MR 2013;34:525–34.
70. Herbert A, Walters MT, Cawley MI, et al. Lymphocytic interstitial pneumonia identified as lymphoma of mucosa associated lymphoid tissue. J Pathol 1985;146: 129–38.

71. Kradin RL, Mark EJ. Benign lymphoid disorders of the lung, with a theory regarding their development. Hum Pathol 1983;14:857–67.
72. Swigris JJ, Berry GJ, Raffin TA, et al. Lymphoid interstitial pneumonia: a narrative review. Chest 2002;122:2150–64.

# Determining Respiratory Impairment in Connective Tissue Disease–Associated Interstitial Lung Disease

Deborah Assayag, MDCM, FRCPC[a],*,
Christopher J. Ryerson, MD, FRCPC[b]

## KEYWORDS

- Connective tissue disease • Interstitial lung disease • Respiratory impairment
- Pulmonary function testing • Diagnosis

## KEY POINTS

- ILD is a common complication of CTD that has unique management and a poor prognosis.
- Patients with CTD without known pulmonary disease should undergo regular symptom assessment and physical examination for findings suggestive of ILD or other respiratory involvement.
- A comprehensive evaluation for ILD in patients with high-risk features or suggestive findings should include symptom assessment, physical examination, pulmonary function tests, and chest imaging (plain chest radiography or high-resolution computed tomography).
- Clinical, physiologic, and radiologic findings should be integrated in a multidisciplinary setting to guide diagnosis and management.

## INTRODUCTION

Connective tissue diseases (CTDs) include several systemic disorders that frequently result in pulmonary involvement. CTDs can affect the lungs through diseases of the chest wall, pleura, vasculature, airways, and parenchyma. A large percentage of patients with CTD develop interstitial lung disease (ILD), a group of typically progressive and irreversible diseases that are characterized by inflammation or fibrosis of the lung parenchyma.

A diagnosis of ILD in a patient with CTD is associated with significantly increased morbidity and mortality. Dyspnea, the major symptom of ILD, is an important and

Disclosures: None.
[a] Department of Medicine, McGill University, 3755 Cote-Ste-Catherine, G-200, Montreal, Quebec H3T 1E2, Canada; [b] Department of Medicine, St. Paul's Hospital, University of British Columbia, Ward 8B, 1081 Burrard Street, Vancouver, British Columbia V6Z 1Y6, Canada
* Corresponding author.
*E-mail address:* Deborah.assayag@mail.mcgill.ca

Rheum Dis Clin N Am 41 (2015) 213–223
http://dx.doi.org/10.1016/j.rdc.2014.12.003          rheumatic.theclinics.com
0889-857X/15/$ – see front matter © 2015 Elsevier Inc. All rights reserved.

independent predictor of physical function and well-being in patients with CTD-associated ILD (CTD-ILD).[1] ILD is the most common cause of death in patients with systemic sclerosis (SSc)[2] and the inflammatory myopathies.[3] In patients with Sjögren syndrome, any respiratory involvement is associated with reduced quality of life and a four-fold increased risk of death.[4] Early recognition of ILD is therefore important to help guide management and improve prognostication.

This article discusses the approach to the evaluation of respiratory impairment in patients with CTD. We focus specifically on the initial evaluation of ILD in patients with CTD, and summarize the evidence that guides the diagnostic work-up of suspected CTD-ILD.

## PULMONARY INVOLVEMENT IN CONNECTIVE TISSUE DISEASE

Pulmonary symptoms in patients with CTD are nonspecific and can be secondary to pulmonary or nonpulmonary causes. Nonpulmonary causes of dyspnea in patients with CTD include anemia, chest wall disease, and cardiopericardial disease. Pulmonary symptoms can also be related to treatment of the underlying CTD, including drug-induced ILD and opportunistic infections or malignancy that have increased frequency in patients who are chronically immunosuppressed. These nonpulmonary manifestations of CTD and complications of CTD therapy are important to identify because these have unique therapies and often clear benefit from appropriate management.

Dyspnea and cough are also common symptoms of the pulmonary manifestations of CTD, including serositis (eg, pleuritis and associated pleural effusions), vascular disease (eg, thromboembolic disease, pulmonary hypertension), airways disease (eg,

| Table 1 | | |
|---|---|---|
| **Type of respiratory involvement and ILD patterns in CTD** | | |
| | **Respiratory Involvement** | |
| **Connective Tissue Disease** | **Frequent Non-ILD Diseases** | **Frequent ILD Patterns** |
| Rheumatoid arthritis | Pleuritis/pleural effusion<br>Pulmonary nodules<br>Bronchiolitis | UIP, NSIP, OP, LIP, DAD |
| Systemic sclerosis | Pulmonary hypertension<br>Ventilatory restriction from skin<br>  sclerosis<br>Bronchiolitis | NSIP, UIP, OP |
| Sjögren syndrome | Bronchiolitis<br>Pulmonary amyloidosis<br>Pulmonary lymphoma | LIP, NSIP, OP, UIP |
| Inflammatory myopathies | Respiratory muscle weakness<br>Pulmonary hypertension | NSIP, OP, UIP, DAD |
| Mixed connective tissue disease | Pulmonary hypertension<br>Pleuritis/pleural effusion<br>Thromboembolic disease | NSIP, OP, UIP |
| Systemic lupus erythematosus | Pleuritis/pleural effusion<br>Diffuse alveolar hemorrhage<br>Diaphragmatic dysfunction<br>  (shrinking lung syndrome)<br>Pulmonary hypertension<br>Thromboembolic disease | NSIP, DAD, OP |

*Abbreviations:* DAD, diffuse alveolar hemorrhage; LIP, lymphocytic interstitial pneumonia; NSIP, nonspecific interstitial pneumonia; OP, organizing pneumonia; UIP, usual interstitial pneumonia.

follicular or obliterative bronchiolitis), and ILD (**Table 1**). Each CTD is associated with multiple pulmonary manifestations; however, different CTD subtypes predispose to specific patterns of pulmonary involvement. ILD is most common in patients with rheumatoid arthritis (RA), SSc, the inflammatory myopathies, Sjögren syndrome, and mixed CTD, but occurs at a lower frequency in systemic lupus erythematosus. Similarly, each CTD predisposes to specific ILD subtypes. Nonspecific interstitial pneumonia is the most common pattern in most CTD-ILDs, but other patterns are frequently observed, including usual interstitial pneumonia (UIP), organizing pneumonia, diffuse alveolar damage, and lymphocytic interstitial pneumonia.

## EVALUATION FOR INTERSTITIAL LUNG DISEASE IN CONNECTIVE TISSUE DISEASE

The extent of evaluation for ILD in patients with CTD should be based on the pretest likelihood of ILD. In patients with CTD with a high probability of ILD, a comprehensive initial evaluation should include clinical, physiologic, and radiologic evaluations. This can often distinguish between ILD and non-ILD pulmonary involvement (**Table 2**). Patients with a low probability of ILD should still undergo regular screening including symptom assessment and physical examination, but may not require detailed physiologic or radiologic studies.

### Symptom Assessment and Physical Examination

Patients with CTD should routinely be questioned regarding the presence of dyspnea, because it is typically the first and predominant symptom of ILD. Dyspnea is a significant predictor of physical function, fatigue, psychological well-being, and global functioning in CTD-ILD, even after adjusting for the severity of lung involvement.[1] Dyspnea can be quantified using detailed questionnaires[5]; however, these questionnaires are typically time consuming and none are validated in CTD-ILD. In a clinical setting,

**Table 2**
**Common findings of respiratory involvement in CTD**

| | ILD | Non-ILD Respiratory Disease | | |
| | | Airways Disease | Pleural Disease | Pulmonary Hypertension |
| --- | --- | --- | --- | --- |
| Symptoms and physical examination | Dyspnea Crackles | Dyspnea Wheezing | Dyspnea Pain Decreased breath sounds | Dyspnea Loud P2 Right heart insufficiency |
| Chest imaging | Decreased lung volumes Reticulation Traction bronchiectasis Ground glass opacities Honeycombing | Air trapping Hyperinflation Airway wall thickening Centrilobular nodularity Normal parenchyma | Effusion Pleural thickening Atelectasis | Enlarged pulmonary arteries Dilated right ventricle Mosaic perfusion Centrilobular ground glass nodules |
| PFT | Restrictive pattern Low D$_{LCO}$ | Obstructive or mixed pattern Normal or low D$_{LCO}$ | Restrictive pattern Normal D$_{LCO}$ | Low D$_{LCO}$ Normal flow rates and lung volumes |

Abbreviations: D$_{LCO}$, diffusion capacity of the lung for carbon monoxide; PFT, pulmonary function test.

dyspnea and associated functional limitation can be quickly assessed and quantified using the Modified Medical Research Council scale (ranging from 0 to 4, where 0 is breathless on strenuous exercise, and 4 is too breathless to leave the house).[6] The Modified Medical Research Council scale, initially developed and validated in patients with chronic obstructive pulmonary disease, is associated with activity limitation, anxiety, and depression in ILD.[7,8] The Modified Medical Research Council scale is not validated in CTD-ILD, but is likely an appropriate screening tool that can be used as a baseline measurement to identify worsening dyspnea and function over time. Other symptoms commonly reported in patients with CTD-ILD include cough, sputum production, and fatigue.[9] Patients that develop these nonspecific symptoms without a clear cause should undergo a detailed evaluation for CTD-ILD.

All patients with CTD should undergo a thorough physical examination for features of ILD at baseline and this should be repeated at regular follow-up visits. The most common examination feature of ILD is crackles on auscultation. Auscultatory crackles can precede the development of clinically apparent symptoms[10] and should prompt further investigations when identified.[11] Tachypnea, hypoxemia, and reduced chest wall expansion can be observed, but are more typical of advanced ILD. Digital clubbing can occur in CTD-ILD, but is less common than in idiopathic pulmonary fibrosis (IPF).[12,13]

### Pulmonary Function Tests

Pulmonary function tests (PFTs) are used to screen patients with CTD for ILD, to support a new diagnosis in patients with suspected CTD-ILD, or to monitor disease activity and progression in patients with an established CTD-ILD diagnosis. PFTs should be performed in all patients with unexplained symptoms or physical examination findings that are consistent with ILD. However, PFTs can be normal in early ILD, and thus the presence of normal physiology does not rule out mild ILD in patients with a high pretest probability. A normal PFT can also indicate the presence of ILD if previous measurements showed supranormal values, illustrating the importance of comparison with previous tests.

Reduced diffusion capacity of the lung for carbon monoxide ($D_{LCO}$) is often the first physiologic manifestation of ILD,[14] but this is not specific for ILD and pulmonary vascular disease can present with similar findings. More advanced ILD is characterized by a restrictive pattern with proportionately reduced flow rates (forced vital capacity [FVC] and forced expiratory volume in 1 second), reduced lung volumes (total lung capacity), and reduced $D_{LCO}$.[14,15] Once a diagnosis of ILD is established, repeated testing at regular intervals should be performed to quantify the severity of the impairment, assess for disease progression, and monitor response to treatment. A 5% to 10% decline in the FVC is considered clinically important in IPF[16] and this is likely a reasonable threshold to indicate worsening ILD in patients with CTD-ILD.

### Functional Assessment

Functional assessment is most often performed in patients with ILD by measuring the six-minute-walk distance (6MWD) or less commonly using a cardiopulmonary exercise test. The 6MWD is a standardized tool that provides a simple measure of functional capacity and may add prognostic information beyond standard PFTs.[17] The 6MWD correlates with ILD severity (PFT measurements) and quality of life in SSc,[18,19] and both the baseline and change in 6MWD are independent predictors of mortality in IPF.[20] The major limitation of the 6MWD in CTD-ILD is the lack of organ specificity, because abnormalities can also be caused by cardiac disease, pulmonary hypertension, and musculoskeletal disease.[18] In addition, patients with significant peripheral vascular involvement (eg, Raynaud phenomenon) often require pulse oximetry via a forehead or earlobe saturation probe and this equipment can be unreliable and is not universally available. Despite its limitations in identifying ILD in patients with CTD, the 6MWD can be used to monitor disease progression and provide prognostic information in patients with established CTD-ILD.

Cardiopulmonary exercise testing provides a global assessment of the systems involved in exercise and is typically performed in the evaluation of undiagnosed dyspnea. Cardiopulmonary exercise testing can be useful in CTD-ILD to determine if the dyspnea is primarily caused by ILD (ie, ventilatory limitation to exercise with associated hypoxemia),[21] pulmonary vascular disease, cardiac disease, or some other etiology.[22,23]

### Chest Imaging

Plain chest radiography lacks sensitivity and specificity for ILD in a screening setting[24] but may still be useful in the initial evaluation of pulmonary symptoms in CTD because it can identify ILD and other CTD-associated pulmonary manifestations (eg, pleural effusions or pneumonia). High-resolution computed tomography (HRCT) can be used to reliably diagnose or exclude ILD; however, it is costly and associated with nontrivial radiation exposure that increases the risk of malignancy.[25] HRCT is thus not routinely used as a serial screening test in asymptomatic patients with CTD. HRCT of the chest is essential in patients with suspected ILD, and is more sensitive than plain radiography in diagnosing ILD.[24] HRCT can also guide management by suggesting the ILD subtype and providing prognostic information. A radiologic pattern of UIP (subpleural, lower lung–predominant reticulation, traction bronchiectasis, and honeycombing with an absence of ground glass or nodularity) is highly specific for histopathologic UIP in patients with RA,[26] and is associated with a poor prognosis.[27] The extent of fibrosis on HRCT also suggests a poor prognosis in multiple CTD-ILD subtypes,[28–30] and can provide further evidence of stability or worsening in patients with unclear evidence of progression.

### Bronchoscopy and Surgical Lung Biopsy

Bronchoalveolar lavage has no clear role in establishing the diagnosis of CTD-ILD,[31] although it can be helpful to exclude infection, diffuse alveolar hemorrhage, and other causes of ILD in patients with an unclear diagnosis. Transbronchial biopsy has low sensitivity and specificity for diagnosing CTD-ILD and should be discouraged outside of specific situations (eg, patients with suspected sarcoidosis).

Surgical lung biopsy permits a more detailed evaluation of the lung histopathology and is able to identify specific CTD-ILD subtypes. Surgical lung biopsy is particularly useful in cases where the diagnosis of CTD is not yet established, or if a competing diagnosis is possible. Some histopathologic features make the diagnosis of CTD-ILD more likely, including the presence of lymphoid aggregates, interstitial fibrosis with overlapping patterns, bronchiolocentricity, lack of well-formed granulomas, and the presence of rheumatoid nodules.[32] Lung biopsies with any of these findings should prompt a detailed assessment for an occult CTD. Surgical lung biopsy is generally not performed in patients with established CTD given the significant risk of complications and the current lack of evidence that the histopathologic pattern should influence management of CTD-ILD.

### INTEGRATING DATA TO GUIDE THERAPY: MULTIDISCIPLINARY EVALUATION

The data described previously should be synthesized to guide management. Central to this process is a multidisciplinary team that includes a rheumatologist, respirologist, thoracic radiologist, and lung pathologist. This team is critical to determining the relative benefits and risks of therapy, based on the burden of disease, risk of progression, expected response to therapy, and likelihood of adverse effects.

## FOLLOW-UP EVALUATION

There is no evidence to guide how often patients with CTD should be screened for ILD or how often patients with CTD with existing ILD should be monitored for disease progression. Patients with CTD without known ILD should have at least annual clinical assessment for development of ILD, usually consisting of symptom assessment and physical examination, with supplemental information provided by physiologic, functional, and radiologic evaluation in cases with suggestive findings or high-risk features. Patients with CTD with existing ILD are typically evaluated every 6 months, with more or less frequent evaluation depending on the overall prognosis and risk of ILD progression.

Older age, male sex, and severity of lung function impairment are consistently associated with increased mortality in RA-ILD and SSc-ILD,[33,34] and these variables are included in a clinical prediction model that accurately predicts mortality in patients with CTD-ILD.[35] Longitudinal data (eg, decline in FVC, worsening HRCT fibrosis) can provide additional prognostic information. As described previously, these data can be synthesized in a multidisciplinary setting to identify patients with progressive disease who may require frequent follow-up and more aggressive therapy.

## DISCUSSION

The optimal method for determining respiratory impairment in patients with CTD is unknown because of an absence of high-quality data in this population. Recommendations for the evaluation and management of CTD-ILD are thus primarily based on expert opinion that is derived from clinical experience or extrapolation from evidence in other ILDs. We propose the algorithm presented in **Fig. 1** to guide the evaluation of possible ILD in patients with CTD; however, there remain several unanswered questions.

### Can We Reliably Predict Which Patients with Connective Tissue Disease Will Develop Interstitial Lung Disease?

It is difficult to predict which patients with CTD will develop ILD and which of these will progress to clinically significant disease that requires therapy. Some asymptomatic patients have abnormal pulmonary function and early ILD,[36] suggesting that there may be a role for ILD screening in asymptomatic individuals. This could be performed using spirometry or D$_{LCO}$ measurements. However, these are generally limited and costly resources that are not ideal for regular screening in a large population. Other strategies are therefore necessary to further narrow the population that requires targeted screening.

Several risk factors for ILD have been identified in patients with CTD; however, the clinical utility of these is unknown. Demographic predictors of ILD in patients with CTD include older age and male sex. The presence of certain autoantibodies is also associated with increased risk of ILD (eg, anticyclic citrullinated peptides in RA and Scl-70 in SSc).[37,38] Additional biomarkers that are associated with the presence or severity of CTD-ILD include Krebs von den lungen-6,[33,39] CC chemokine ligand 18,[40] and surfactant protein D.[41] Despite these associations, there is currently no evidence that patients with high-risk clinical features should undergo more rigorous serial screening for ILD. Additional studies are therefore needed to validate predictors of ILD onset and to determine the role for these predictors in clinical practice.

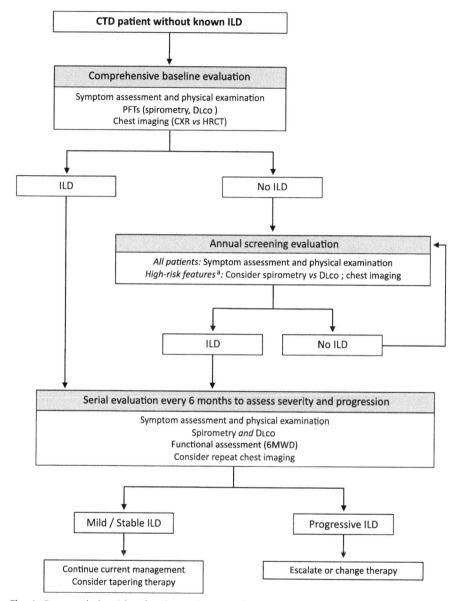

**Fig. 1.** Proposed algorithm for the evaluation of ILD in patients with CTD. [a] High-risk features can include demographic features (eg, increased age, male sex), CTD subtype (eg, diffuse cutaneous SSc), autoantibody status (positive anti–Scl-70 antibody), and others. CXR, plain chest radiography.

### What Changes Should Prompt Escalation of Therapy in Connective Tissue Disease–Interstitial Lung Disease?

ILD progression can be measured by symptoms, physiology, or radiology. However, it is not clear what constitutes a minimum clinically important difference (MCID) for each of these domains. There is no reliable threshold for a clinically meaningful change in subjectively reported dyspnea. The MCID has been reported in other populations for several standardized dyspnea questionnaires. However, these questionnaires are not typically used in a clinical setting, have not been validated in CTD-ILD, and their MCIDs in CTD-ILD are unknown. Similarly, the MCID for physiologic change is uncertain, although there are data from other ILD populations that can likely be extrapolated to CTD-ILD. In patients with IPF, an absolute decline of 5% to 10% in the FVC is considered clinically significant.[16] This magnitude of decline is likely also meaningful in CTD-ILD. However, CTD-ILD often progresses less rapidly than IPF, and thus fewer patients with CTD-ILD meet this relatively high threshold of change during a single follow-up interval. It is unknown whether smaller changes in FVC are meaningful in CTD-ILD, and particularly if serial small declines in FVC are significant. There are no data on the MCID for radiologic findings and, similar to dyspnea, these changes are typically reported in a subjective manner in clinical practice that prevents a quantitative comparison among serial studies.

Patients can have progression in any one or in all three of these domains, and it is challenging to confidently identify progression in individuals with borderline or inconsistent findings. Patients with progression in at least two of these three domains are generally considered to have had ILD progression, although there are some exceptions to this rule (eg, respiratory muscle weakness can worsen both dyspnea and physiology in the absence of ILD progression). Patients with borderline changes in all domains, and patients with change in only one domain, have uncertain findings that may prompt short-interval reassessment or further evaluation with functional assessment.

### Should the Approach to Management Be the Same for All Connective Tissue Disease–Interstitial Lung Disease Subtypes?

CTDs are associated with several underlying ILD subtypes, most often including nonspecific interstitial pneumonia, UIP, and organizing pneumonia. The ILD subtype provides important prognostic information, specifically with UIP having worse prognosis than non-UIP patterns in RA-ILD and some other CTD-ILD subtypes.[27,42] However, it is unclear whether the approach to management should also differ among these subtypes.

Most CTD-ILD subtypes are managed with systemic immunosuppressive medications, regardless of the underlying ILD pattern. Recent studies have shown lack of benefit and significant harm from immunosuppressive medications in IPF (ie, idiopathic UIP),[43] but it is unknown whether these therapies have similar deleterious effects in UIP associated with CTD. Future studies of treatment in CTD-ILD should stratify patients according to their ILD pattern (ie, UIP vs non-UIP) to determine whether treatment strategies should differ among ILD subtypes, and specifically whether immunosuppressive therapies are beneficial in CTD-associated UIP. The role of histopathologic evaluation in CTD-ILD would increase if therapeutic responses were found to differ according to ILD subtype.

### SUMMARY

ILD and other forms of respiratory involvement are common in CTDs. The evaluation for lung disease in patients with CTD at high risk of ILD should be comprehensive and include at least annual clinical, physiologic, and radiologic assessment. Patients with a low pretest probability of ILD may require only intermittent screening with a symptom assessment and physical examination. The data gathered during the evaluation for CTD-ILD should be integrated using a multidisciplinary approach to determine the most appropriate management for each patient. Additional studies are needed to clarify how and how often patients with CTD should be screened for ILD, whether there are features that can reliably identify high-risk patients, what monitoring should be performed in patients with established ILD, and how findings should be integrated to guide management.

## REFERENCES

1. Swigris JJ, Yorke J, Sprunger DB, et al. Assessing dyspnea and its impact on patients with connective tissue disease-related interstitial lung disease. Respir Med 2010;104:1350–5.
2. Steen VD, Medsger TA. Changes in causes of death in systemic sclerosis, 1972-2002. Ann Rheum Dis 2007;66:940–4.
3. Cottin V, Thivolet-Bejui F, Reynaud-Gaubert M, et al. Interstitial lung disease in amyopathic dermatomyositis, dermatomyositis and polymyositis. Eur Respir J 2003;22:245–50.
4. Palm O, Garen T, Berge Enger T, et al. Clinical pulmonary involvement in primary Sjogren's syndrome: prevalence, quality of life and mortality: a retrospective study based on registry data. Rheumatology (Oxford) 2013;52:173–9.
5. Parshall MB, Schwartzstein RM, Adams L, et al. An official American Thoracic Society statement: update on the mechanisms, assessment, and management of dyspnea. Am J Respir Crit Care Med 2012;185:435–52.
6. Papiris SA, Daniil ZD, Malagari K, et al. The Medical Research Council dyspnea scale in the estimation of disease severity in idiopathic pulmonary fibrosis. Respir Med 2005;99:755–61.
7. Kozu R, Jenkins S, Senjyu H. Evaluation of activity limitation in patients with idiopathic pulmonary fibrosis grouped according to medical research council dyspnea grade. Arch Phys Med Rehabil 2014;95:950–5.
8. Holland AE, Fiore JF Jr, Bell EC, et al. Dyspnoea and comorbidity contribute to anxiety and depression in interstitial lung disease. Respirology 2014;9:1215–21.
9. Pan L, Liu Y, Sun R, et al. Comparison of characteristics of connective tissue disease-associated interstitial lung diseases, undifferentiated connective tissue disease-associated interstitial lung diseases, and idiopathic pulmonary fibrosis in Chinese Han population: a retrospective study. Clin Dev Immunol 2013;2013:121578.
10. Gochuico Br, Avila NA, Chow CK, et al. Progressive preclinical interstitial lung disease in rheumatoid arthritis. Arch Intern Med 2008;168:159–66.
11. Cordier JF, Cottin V. Neglected evidence in idiopathic pulmonary fibrosis: from history to earlier diagnosis. Eur Respir J 2013;42:916–23.
12. Rajasekaran A, Shovlin D, Saravanan V, et al. Interstitial lung disease in patients with rheumatoid arthritis: comparison with cryptogenic fibrosing alveolitis over 5 years. J Rheumatol 2006;33:1250–3.
13. Ishioka S, Nakamura K, Maeda A, et al. Clinical evaluation of idiopathic interstitial pneumonia and interstitial pneumonia associated with collagen vascular disease using logistic regression analysis. Intern Med 2000;39:213–9.
14. Nogueira CR, Nápolis LM, Bagatin E, et al. Lung diffusing capacity relates better to short-term progression on HRCT abnormalities than spirometry in mild asbestosis. Am J Ind Med 2011;54:185–93.
15. Pellegrino R, Viegi G, Brusasco V, et al. Interpretative strategies for lung function tests. Eur Respir J 2005;26:948–68.
16. Raghu G, Collard HR, Egan JJ, et al. An official ATS/ERS/JRS/ALAT statement: idiopathic pulmonary fibrosis: evidence-based guidelines for diagnosis and management. Am J Respir Crit Care Med 2011;183:788–824.

17. ATS Committee on Proficiency Standards for Clinical Pulmonary Function Laboratories. ATS statement: guidelines for the six-minute walk test. Am J Respir Crit Care Med 2002;166:111–7.

18. Deuschle K, Weinert K, Becker MO, et al. Six-minute walk distance as a marker for disability and complaints in patients with systemic sclerosis. Clin Exp Rheumatol 2011;29:S53–9.

19. Schoindre Y, Meune C, Dinh-Xuan AT, et al. Lack of specificity of the 6-minute walk test as an outcome measure for patients with systemic sclerosis. J Rheumatol 2009;36:1481–5.

20. du Bois RM, Albera C, Bradford WZ, et al. 6-Minute walk distance is an independent predictor of mortality in patients with idiopathic pulmonary fibrosis. Eur Respir J 2014;43:1421–9.

21. Ross RM. ATS/ACCP statement on cardiopulmonary exercise testing. Am J Respir Crit Care Med 2003;167:211–77.

22. Dumitrescu D, Oudiz RJ, Karpouzas G, et al. Developing pulmonary vasculopathy in systemic sclerosis, detected with non-invasive cardiopulmonary exercise testing. PLoS One 2010;5:e14293.

23. Armstrong HF, Thirapatarapong W, Dussault NE, et al. Distinguishing pulmonary hypertension in interstitial lung disease by ventilation and perfusion defects measured by cardiopulmonary exercise testing. Respiration 2013;86:407–13.

24. Mathieson JR, Mayo JR, Staples CA, et al. Chronic diffuse infiltrative lung disease: comparison of diagnostic accuracy of CT and chest radiography. Radiology 1989;171:111–6.

25. van der Bruggen-Bogaarts BA, Broerse JJ, Lammers JW, et al. Radiation exposure in standard and high-resolution chest CT scans. Chest 1995;107:113–5.

26. Assayag D, Elicker BM, Urbania TH, et al. Rheumatoid arthritis-associated interstitial lung disease: radiologic identification of usual interstitial pneumonia pattern. Radiology 2014;270:583–8.

27. Kim EJ, Elicker BM, Maldonado F, et al. Usual interstitial pneumonia in rheumatoid arthritis-associated interstitial lung disease. Eur Respir J 2010;35:1322–8.

28. Kocheril SV, Appleton BE, Somers EC, et al. Comparison of disease progression and mortality of connective tissue disease-related interstitial lung disease and idiopathic interstitial pneumonia. Arthritis Care Res 2005;53:549–57.

29. Walsh SL, Sverzellati N, Devaraj A, et al. Connective tissue disease related fibrotic lung disease: high resolution computed tomographic and pulmonary function indices as prognostic determinants. Thorax 2014;69:216–22.

30. Goh NS, Desai SR, Veeraraghavan S, et al. Interstitial lung disease in systemic sclerosis: a simple staging system. Am J Respir Crit Care Med 2008;177:1248–54.

31. Kowal-Bielecka O, Kowal K, Chyczewska E. Utility of bronchoalveolar lavage in evaluation of patients with connective tissue diseases. Clin Chest Med 2010;31:423–31.

32. Urisman A, Jones KD. Pulmonary pathology in connective tissue disease. Semin Respir Crit Care Med 2014;35:201–12.

33. Winstone TA, Assayag D, Wilcox PG, et al. Predictors of mortality and progression in scleroderma-associated interstitial lung disease: a systematic review. Chest 2014;146:422–36.

34. Assayag D, Lubin M, Lee JS, et al. Predictors of mortality in rheumatoid arthritis-related interstitial lung disease. Respirology 2014;19:493–500.

35. Ryerson CJ, Vittinghoff E, Ley B, et al. Predicting survival across chronic interstitial lung disease: the ILD-gap model. Chest 2014;145:723–8.

36. Chen J, Shi Y, Wang X, et al. Asymptomatic preclinical rheumatoid arthritis-associated interstitial lung disease. Clin Dev Immunol 2013;2013:406927.
37. Kelly CA, Saravanan V, Nisar M, et al. Rheumatoid arthritis-related interstitial lung disease: associations, prognostic factors and physiological and radiological characteristics. A large multicentre UK study. Rheumatology (Oxford) 2014;53: 1676–82.
38. Cepeda EJ, Reveille JD. Autoantibodies in systemic sclerosis and fibrosing syndromes: clinical indications and relevance. Curr Opin Rheumatol 2004;16: 723–32.
39. Arai S, Kurasawa K, Maezawa R, et al. Marked increase in serum KL-6 and surfactant protein D levels during the first 4 weeks after treatment predicts poor prognosis in patients with active interstitial pneumonia associated with polymyositis/dermatomyositis. Mod Rheumatol 2013;23:872–83.
40. Tiev KP, Hua-Huy T, Kettaneh A, et al. Serum CC chemokine ligand-18 predicts lung disease worsening in systemic sclerosis. Eur Respir J 2011;38:1355–60.
41. Elhaj M, Charles J, Pedroza C, et al. Can serum surfactant protein D or CC-chemokine ligand 18 predict outcome of interstitial lung disease in patients with early systemic sclerosis? J Rheumatol 2013;40:1114–20.
42. Tsuchiya Y, Takayanagi N, Sugiura H, et al. Lung diseases directly associated with rheumatoid arthritis and their relationship to outcome. Eur Respir J 2011; 37:1411–7.
43. Idiopathic Pulmonary Fibrosis Clinical Research Network, Raghu G, Anstrom KJ, et al. Prednisone, azathioprine, and N-acetylcysteine for pulmonary fibrosis. N Engl J Med 2012;366:1968–77.

# Lung Disease in Rheumatoid Arthritis

Zulma X. Yunt, MD, Joshua J. Solomon, MD*

## KEYWORDS

- Rheumatoid arthritis • Extra-articular disease • Pulmonary • Interstitial lung disease
- Interstitial pneumonia • Bronchiolitis • Pleural effusion • Drug-induced lung disease

## KEY POINTS

- Rheumatoid arthritis commonly affects the lungs and can involve any compartment of the respiratory system.
- Usual interstitial pneumonia and nonspecific interstitial pneumonia are the most common patterns seen with interstitial involvement in rheumatoid arthritis.
- Treatment consists of long-term therapy with immunomodulatory agents.
- Further studies are needed to better characterize patients, predict progression, and determine optimal therapeutic regimens.

## INTRODUCTION

Rheumatoid arthritis (RA) is a progressive, systemic autoimmune disorder characterized by articular and extra-articular manifestations. The lung is commonly a site of extra-articular disease. Within the lung, manifestations of RA vary and may include airways, parenchymal, vascular, and/or pleural disease (**Box 1**). Manifestations of lung disease in RA typically follow the development of articular disease, but in some instances lung involvement is the first manifestation of RA and is the most aggressive feature of the disease.[1] Clinicians should therefore remain alert to the possibility of lung disease in all patients with RA.

## EPIDEMIOLOGY

RA is the most common connective tissue disease (CTD), with a prevalence of 0.5% to 2% in the general population.[2] The disease occurs more frequently in women than in men with a ratio of 3:1. Extra-articular disease occurs in approximately 50% of patients, with the lung being a common site of involvement.[3] Lung involvement may

Disclosure: NIH Diversity Supplement 3R01 HL109517–01A1S1.
Autoimmune Lung Center, National Jewish Health, 1400 Jackson Street, Denver, CO 80206, USA
* Corresponding author.
*E-mail address:* solomonj@njhealth.org

rheumatic.theclinics.com

---

**Box 1**
**Pulmonary manifestation of RA**

**Interstitial lung disease**
- Usual interstitial pneumonia
- Nonspecific interstitial pneumonia
- Organizing pneumonia
- Lymphocytic interstitial pneumonia
- Acute interstitial pneumonia

**Airways disease**
- Follicular bronchiolitis
- Constrictive bronchiolitis (obliterative bronchiolitis)
- Bronchiectasis
- Cricoarytenoid arthritis

Rheumatoid nodules

**Pleural disease**
- Pleuritis
- Pleural effusion
- Pneumothorax
- Empyema

**Vascular disease**
- Pulmonary hypertension
- Vasculitis

**Rheumatoid pneumoconiosis (Caplan syndrome)**

**Drug toxicity**

**Infection**

**Amyloidosis**

**Fibrobullous disease**

---

occur in as many as 67% of patients, although some reports indicate a lower incidence (around 10%–20%).[4–6] This wide variation reflects differences in study design, study populations, and the way that lung disease in RA is defined. Many patients with RA have no clinical symptoms of respiratory disease despite radiographic or physiologic evidence of lung abnormalities, often leading to a misrepresentation of disease prevalence. In a study of 52 patients with RA, high-resolution computed tomography (HRCT) abnormalities were identified in 67.3% with only 40% of patients having respiratory symptoms.[4] In addition to respiratory involvement from RA, medication toxicity and secondary pulmonary infections are important sources of lung disease that must be considered in patients with RA.

Mortality is increased in patients with RA with extra-articular manifestations relative to those without extra-articular involvement, with cardiovascular disease, infection, and lung disease being the leading causes. Mortality in RA is greatest within the first 5 to 7 years after diagnosis and risk may be slightly higher in men than in women, with a mortality ratio of 2.07:1.97 respectively.[7,8] Lung disease alone accounts for 10% to 20% of deaths in patients with RA, and most of these are attributed to interstitial lung disease (ILD).[9–11]

## FORMS OF LUNG DISEASE IN RHEUMATOID ARTHRITIS
### Interstitial Lung Disease

ILD refers to heterogeneous group of parenchymal lung disorders classified by distinct clinical, pathologic, and radiographic features. The 2013 American Thoracic Society/European Respiratory Society official classification of the idiopathic interstitial pneumonias (IIPs) outlines the most recent histopathologic classifications of ILD, many of which may be seen in RA.[12] The most common forms of ILD associated with RA are usual interstitial pneumonia (UIP) and nonspecific interstitial pneumonia (NSIP); however, organizing pneumonia (OP), desquamative interstitial pneumonia, lymphocytic interstitial pneumonia, diffuse alveolar damage, and acute interstitial pneumonia have been reported.[13,14] Smoking, advanced age, high-titer anticyclic citrullinated peptide antibodies, high-titer rheumatoid factor, family history of RA, and in some studies male gender are all risk factors for developing RA-ILD.[15]

### Pathophysiology

The pathophysiologic basis for development of ILD in patients with RA remains elusive. Available data suggest a role for both environmental and genetic factors. Specific human leukocyte antigen (HLA) variants including HLA-B54, HLA-DQB1*0601, HLA-B40, and HLA-DR4 have been associated with RA-ILD.[16–19] Similarly, cigarette smoking has been linked with both RA and RA-ILD.[20,21] Some speculate that the lungs may be a site of initial immune dysregulation that leads to the development of RA.[22] Citrullinated proteins have been identified in bronchoalveolar lavage fluid from cigarette smokers without RA, and RA-related autoantibodies are detectable in the sputum of patients identified to be at risk for RA.[23,24]

It is hoped that investigations of biomarkers for RA-ILD will identify key molecules and thus provide more insight into disease immunopathogenesis and avenues for early diagnosis. To date, serum autoantibodies against multiple citrullinated proteins and peptides including fibrinogen, vimentin, and citrullinated isoforms of heat shock protein 90 and matrix metalloproteinase-7 (MMP-7) and interferon-gamma inducible protein 10[25–27] have been associated with RA-ILD. The precise role of these proteins in tissue-specific disease manifestations is not known.

### Prognosis and mortality

Information pertaining to the natural history of RA-ILD relies on data from a limited number of studies and more data are needed to confidently characterize prognosis and mortality within this population. The available studies indicate that patients with RA-ILD have a 3-fold increased risk of death relative to those without ILD. In addition, although overall mortality from RA seems to be decreasing, mortality from RA-ILD seems to be increasing, particularly in women and in older age groups.[28,29] A study of 582 patients with RA identified a median survival of 2.6 years in those with ILD compared with 10 years in age-matched patients with RA without ILD.[29] Within the category of RA-ILD, prognosis varies significantly depending on the precise histopathologic form of RA-ILD and from patient to patient. UIP is the most common subtype of RA-ILD and carries the worst prognosis,[1,14,30] which differs from CTDs overall, in which the most common pattern of ILD is NSIP.[1] High-quality studies of additional factors that influence prognosis are lacking. A recent systematic review of current literature investigating predictors of mortality in RA-ILD included 10 studies and found that male gender, older age, lower lung diffusion capacity for carbon monoxide (DLCO), a finding of UIP, and the extent of fibrosis were significant predictors of mortality.[31]

### Clinical features

Exertional dyspnea and cough of insidious onset are the predominant clinical symptoms of RA-ILD. Fatigue and generalized weakness are also frequently seen. Radiographic evidence of ILD on HRCT precedes the development of respiratory symptoms in a significant number of patients with RA and time to development of symptoms for patients with subclinical ILD is not known. Given the prevalence of lung involvement in RA, clinicians should have a low threshold to pursue evaluation of new respiratory complaints in this population.[20] Once present, symptoms usually progress over time; however, the rate of progression is variable from patient to patient and within the different histopathologic forms of ILD. Studies indicate that patients with UIP may progress faster than other subtypes of ILD in RA and at rates similar to those reported for idiopathic pulmonary fibrosis (IPF).[14,32]

### Radiographic features

HRCT has increased the diagnostic sensitivity and accuracy for RA-ILD greatly compared with chest radiograph alone. In a study of 150 consecutive individuals with RA, HRCT evidence of ILD was seen in 19% of patients; however, bilateral interstitial infiltrates were seen on chest radiograph in less than 3%.[6] The most common radiographic finding is a UIP pattern, which is characterized on HRCT by peripheral basilar predominant reticular abnormalities, honeycombing, traction bronchiectasis, and minimal to no ground-glass opacification (**Fig. 1**). NSIP is the other common pattern in RA-ILD and is characterized by reticulation and ground-glass with little or no architectural distortion or honeycombing (**Fig. 2**).

### Diagnostic evaluation

Early symptoms of respiratory disease, particularly dyspnea on exertion, may be difficult to ascertain in patients with exercise-limiting joint disease. Clinicians should therefore remain alert to subtle symptoms, including new cough, change in activity level, or low resting oxygen levels. The initial diagnostic evaluation for patients with RA with respiratory symptoms includes an assessment of lung physiology with pulmonary function tests (PFTs), radiographic imaging with HRCT, and assessment of the

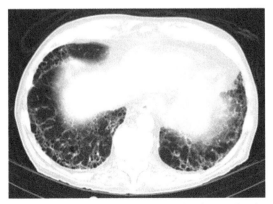

**Fig. 1.** UIP in RA. The UIP pattern consists of peripheral basilar predominant reticular abnormalities, honeycombing, traction bronchiectasis, and minimal to no ground-glass opacification.

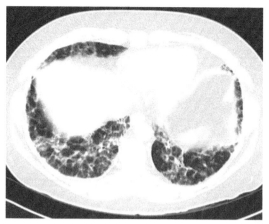

**Fig. 2.** Nonspecific interstitial pneumonia in RA. The nonspecific interstitial pneumonia pattern consists of reticulation and ground-glass with little or no architectural distortion or honeycombing.

patient's oxygenation both at rest and with activity. Initial PFTs should include components of lung volume, airflow with bronchodilator challenge, and DLCO measurements. For initial imaging, HRCT imaging is recommended rather than chest radiograph for its superior sensitivity in detecting early parenchymal disease and small airways disease.[6,33] Lung biopsy is not indicated in most cases of RA-ILD; however, if the diagnosis is uncertain or computed tomography findings are atypical, surgical lung biopsy may be useful. Transbronchial biopsies have low yield and are generally not performed, although they may be helpful for the purpose of ruling out drug-related disease or infection. For all patients with diffuse parenchymal disease, infection and drug-induced disease must be ruled out before making a diagnosis of ILD. Numerous medications used in the treatment of RA have reported pulmonary toxicities (**Table 1**).

*Treatment*
No randomized placebo-controlled therapeutic trials have been performed to date in RA-ILD. As such, no consensus therapeutic guidelines have been established. Our practice is to monitor these patients closely for progression of disease and initiate treatment when clinical symptoms manifest or when there is physiologic evidence of progressive disease. In all cases, risk of therapy must be weighed against threat of disease.

Current treatment regimens usually involve corticosteroid therapy with or without a cytotoxic agent; most commonly azathioprine, mycophenolate mofetil (MMF), or cyclophosphamide. Recent retrospective analyses centered on treatment of RA-ILD with MMF and rituximab have shown promising results. In a study of 125 patients with CTD-related ILD treated with MMF, subgroup analysis of 18 patients with RA-ILD identified a trend toward improved forced vital capacity following initiation of therapy.[34] Further, this drug has shown good patient tolerability and safety in patients with CTD-ILD.[34,35] Retrospective studies with rituximab have recently shown success in cases of refractory CTD-ILD,[36,37] although larger prospective studies are needed to validate these findings in patients with RA-ILD. Limited reports also exist for treatment with cyclosporine, methotrexate, and tumor necrosis factor (TNF) alpha inhibitors.[36–41] Response to therapy in RA-ILD seems to correlate with histopathologic form of disease. As in IIPs, NSIP shows better response to therapy and prognosis than a UIP

**Table 1**
**Lung toxicity of rheumatoid therapies**

| Medication | Symptoms | Radiopathologic Findings | Incidence |
|---|---|---|---|
| Methotrexate | Dyspnea, cough, fever[62] | Common: bilateral interstitial granulomatous infiltrates with ground-glass opacification on chest CT[62] Uncommon: unilateral infiltrates, pleural effusions, reticulonodular disease, hilar lymphadenopathy[63–66] | 0.3%–11.6%[67] Most cases occur within 2 y of drug initiation and may occur after a single dose[68] |
| Anti-TNF | Dyspnea | Aseptic granulomatous pulmonary nodules, both noncaseating and necrotizing[69,70] Accelerated interstitial lung infiltrates[42,43] Bronchospasm[71] | ILD, 0.5%–3%[72] |
| Leflunomide | Dyspnea, fever, cough[73] | Diffuse or patchy ground-glass opacities. Often with septal thickening[74] | ILD, <1%[73] 2-fold increased risk of new ILD seen in those with prior methotrexate use[75] |
| Rituximab | Dyspnea | Acute/subacute OP[76] Acute respiratory distress syndrome[76] | Unknown |
| Sulfasalazine | Dyspnea, cough | Variable. Most commonly, eosinophilic pneumonia and peripheral eosinophilia[77] Interstitial fibrosis[78] | Unknown |
| Tocilizumab | — | OP[79] Exacerbation of ILD[80] Allergic pneumonitis[81] | Unknown |

*Abbreviations:* CT, computed tomography; TNF, tumor necrosis factor.

pattern.[1,14] Note that control of joint disease does not translate to control of lung disease, and optimal management requires a coordinated approach between an experienced pulmonologist and rheumatologist.

All patients with RA-ILD should be encouraged to abstain from smoking. Smoking-related lung disease should be treated if present. Oxygenation should be evaluated during rest, ambulation, and sleep and supplemental oxygen should be prescribed as indicated. Vaccinations for influenza and pneumococcal pneumonia are recommended for all patients. We also recommend prophylaxis against *Pneumocystis jiroveci* pneumonia for all patients on immunosuppressive therapy. In managing the articular manifestations in patients with RA-ILD, methotrexate use should generally be avoided because of well-documented pulmonary toxicity. TNF-alpha inhibitors should be used with caution in these patients following reports of increased rates of lung toxicity with these agents.[42,43] In spite of these reports, a prospective observational study of 367 patients with RA-ILD showed no increase in mortality following treatment with anti-TNF agents compared with standard immunomodulatory agents.[44] Patients with progressive disease should be considered for lung transplant evaluation. Survival rates after transplant for RA-ILD are similar to those for IPF and with significant improvements in quality-of-life scores following transplantation.[45]

### Airways Involvement (Bronchiolitis, Bronchiectasis, and Cricoarytenoid Disease)

Prevalence of airways disease in RA is high; it occurs in 39% to 60% of patients.[46–48] Any part of the airway may be involved, including the large airways (upper and lower) and distal small airways. The most common manifestations are bronchiectasis, bronchiolitis, airway hyperreactivity, and cricoarytenoid arthritis. PFTs and HRCT obtained with expiratory images are useful in making a diagnosis of airways involvement with HRCT, showing greater sensitivity for detection of small airways disease relative to PFTs.[34]

Cricoarytenoid arthritis and bronchiectasis are the most common forms of large airway involvement. Cricoarytenoid abnormalities occur in as many as 75% of patients, although fewer have clinically significant symptoms.[49] Arthritis of the cricoarytenoid joints leads to midline adduction of the vocal cords with resultant hoarseness and in some cases inspiratory stridor. Bronchiectasis, defined as destruction and widening of the large airways, occurs in 16% to 58% of patients with RA.[50,51] Most cases are not clinically significant but, when present, symptoms include cough and sputum production. Treatment of RA patients with known bronchiectasis using a biologic agent has been reported as an independent risk factor for lower respiratory tract infection.[52]

Small airways disease refers to disease involving the distal airways (2 mm in diameter or less). Two forms of small airways disease (follicular bronchiolitis and constrictive bronchiolitis) have been described in association with RA. Follicular bronchiolitis is identified pathologically by the presence of hyperplastic lymphoid follicles with reactive germ cell centers within bronchiole walls. Constrictive bronchiolitis (also referred to as obliterative bronchiolitis) is identified by concentric narrowing of membranous and respiratory bronchioles caused by peribronchiolar inflammation and fibrosis without evidence of lymphoid hyperplasia.[53] There are limited reports regarding disease course and prognosis for RA-associated follicular and constrictive bronchiolitis. Prognosis is thought to be poor; however, in a recent prospective study in CTD-associated bronchiolitis (in which 50% of patients had RA), the forced expiratory volume in 1 second showed stability over time in both forms, suggesting that bronchiolitis associated with CTD may have a less aggressive course than idiopathic disease.[54,55]

### Rheumatoid Nodules

Rheumatoid necrobiotic nodules are pulmonary lesions histologically composed of a central fibrinoid necrotic region surrounded by mononuclear cells, granulation tissue, lymphocytes, plasma cells, and fibroblasts. The nodules may be single or multiple and are typically found in pleural or subpleural regions, occasionally with cavitation.[56,57] Rheumatoid nodules carry good prognosis and may come and go over time. Neoplasm and infection should be ruled out, but once a diagnosis is made no specific therapy is typically required.

### Vascular Disease

Pulmonary arterial hypertension is exceedingly rare in RA. It is more commonly seen in other CTDs such as scleroderma and systemic lupus erythematosis.[58] The most common form of vascular involvement in RA is rheumatoid vasculitis, which is characterized pathologically by the presence of a destructive inflammatory infiltrate within small and medium-sized blood vessel walls. This condition carries significant morbidity and mortality, but primary involvement of the lung is rare.[59]

## Pleural Involvement

Pleuritis and pleural effusions are the most common forms of pleural disease in RA. RA effusions are exudative and sterile, often with low glucose (80%) and low pH (71.4%).[60] A cytologic finding of elongated macrophages and multinucleated giant cells alongside granulomatous debris is pathognomonic for rheumatoid effusions.[61] These findings mirror those in rheumatoid synovitis or rheumatoid nodules. Occasionally, pleural involvement may precede joint disease. Pleural effusions often resolve spontaneously over time. As with rheumatoid lung nodules, infection and malignancy should be considered and ruled out, if appropriate.

## FUTURE CONSIDERATIONS/SUMMARY

RA is a common disorder with a myriad of pulmonary manifestations. Although any compartment of the respiratory system is at risk, the ILDs cause the greatest concern. In its most severe form, affected patients can develop a fibrotic ILD with progression similar to that seen in IPF. Treatment is based on expert opinion and there are no placebo-controlled trials. In order to effectively care for these patients, a better understanding is needed of the link between synovitis and pulmonary disease. Predictors of lung involvement, biomarkers to clinically phenotype patients, and well-designed treatment trials are urgently needed.

## REFERENCES

1. Lee HK, Kim DS, Yoo B, et al. Histopathologic pattern and clinical features of rheumatoid arthritis-associated interstitial lung disease. Chest 2005;127(6):2019–27 [Key Reference].
2. Gabriel SE, Crowson CS, Kremers HM, et al. Survival in rheumatoid arthritis: a population-based analysis of trends over 40 years. Arthritis Rheum 2003;48(1):54–8.
3. Turesson C, O'Fallon WM, Crowson CS, et al. Occurrence of extraarticular disease manifestations is associated with excess mortality in a community based cohort of patients with rheumatoid arthritis. J Rheumatol 2002;29(1):62–7.
4. Bilgici A, Ulusoy H, Kuru O, et al. Pulmonary involvement in rheumatoid arthritis. Rheumatol Int 2005;25(6):429–35.
5. Mori S, Cho I, Koga Y, et al. Comparison of pulmonary abnormalities on high-resolution computed tomography in patients with early versus longstanding rheumatoid arthritis. J Rheumatol 2008;35(8):1513–21.
6. Dawson JK, Fewins HE, Desmond J, et al. Fibrosing alveolitis in patients with rheumatoid arthritis as assessed by high resolution computed tomography, chest radiography, and pulmonary function tests. Thorax 2001;56(8):622–7.
7. Young A, Koduri G, Batley M, et al. Mortality in rheumatoid arthritis. Increased in the early course of disease, in ischaemic heart disease and in pulmonary fibrosis. Rheumatology (Oxford) 2007;46(2):350–7.
8. Thomas E, Symmons DP, Brewster DH, et al. National study of cause-specific mortality in rheumatoid arthritis, juvenile chronic arthritis, and other rheumatic conditions: a 20 year followup study. J Rheumatol 2003;30(5):958–65.
9. Suzuki A, Ohosone Y, Obana M, et al. Cause of death in 81 autopsied patients with rheumatoid arthritis. J Rheumatol 1994;21(1):33–6.
10. Sihvonen S, Korpela M, Laippala P, et al. Death rates and causes of death in patients with rheumatoid arthritis: a population-based study. Scand J Rheumatol 2004;33(4):221–7.

11. Turesson C, Jacobsson L, Bergstrom U. Extra-articular rheumatoid arthritis: prevalence and mortality. Rheumatology (Oxford) 1999;38(7):668–74.
12. Travis WD, Costabel U, Hansell DM, et al. An official American Thoracic Society/European Respiratory Society statement: update of the international multidisciplinary classification of the idiopathic interstitial pneumonias. Am J Respir Crit Care Med 2013;188(6):733–48.
13. Nakamura Y, Suda T, Kaida Y, et al. Rheumatoid lung disease: prognostic analysis of 54 biopsy-proven cases. Respir Med 2012;106(8):1164–9.
14. Kim EJ, Elicker BM, Maldonado F, et al. Usual interstitial pneumonia in rheumatoid arthritis-associated interstitial lung disease. Eur Respir J 2010;35(6):1322–8 [Key Reference].
15. Solomon JJ, Brown KK. Rheumatoid arthritis-associated interstitial lung disease. Open Access Rheumatol Res Rev 2012;(4):21–31.
16. Charles PJ, Sweatman MC, Markwick JR, et al. HLA-B40: a marker for susceptibility to lung disease in rheumatoid arthritis. Dis Markers 1991;9(2):97–101 [Key Reference].
17. Scott TE, Wise RA, Hochberg MC, et al. HLA-DR4 and pulmonary dysfunction in rheumatoid arthritis. Am J Med 1987;82(4):765–71 [Key Reference].
18. Hillarby MC, McMahon MJ, Grennan DM, et al. HLA associations in subjects with rheumatoid arthritis and bronchiectasis but not with other pulmonary complications of rheumatoid disease. Br J Rheumatol 1993;32(9):794–7 [Key Reference].
19. Sugiyama Y, Ohno S, Kano S, et al. Diffuse panbronchiolitis and rheumatoid arthritis: a possible correlation with HLA-B54. Intern Med 1994;33(10):612–4 [Key Reference].
20. Gochuico BR, Avila NA, Chow CK, et al. Progressive preclinical interstitial lung disease in rheumatoid arthritis. Arch Intern Med 2008;168(2):159–66 [Key Reference].
21. Albano SA, Santana-Sahagun E, Woicman MH. Cigarette smoking and rheumatoid arthritis. Semin Arthritis Rheum 2001;31(3):146–59.
22. Demoruelle MK, Deane KD, Holers VM. When and where does inflammation begin in rheumatoid arthritis? Curr Opin Rheumatol 2014;26(1):64–71.
23. Makrygiannakis D, Hermansson M, Ulfgren AK, et al. Smoking increases peptidylarginine deiminase 2 enzyme expression in human lungs and increases citrullination in BAL cells. Ann Rheum Dis 2008;67(10):1488–92 [Key Reference].
24. Willis VC, Demoruelle MK, Derber LA, et al. Sputum autoantibodies in patients with established rheumatoid arthritis and subjects at risk of future clinically apparent disease. Arthritis Rheum 2013;65(10):2545–54.
25. Harlow L, Rosas IO, Gochuico BR, et al. Identification of citrullinated hsp90 isoforms as novel autoantigens in rheumatoid arthritis-associated interstitial lung disease. Arthritis Rheum 2013;65(4):869–79.
26. Giles JT, Danoff SK, Sokolove J, et al. Association of fine specificity and repertoire expansion of anticitrullinated peptide antibodies with rheumatoid arthritis associated interstitial lung disease. Ann Rheum Dis 2014;73(8):1487–94.
27. Chen J, Doyle TJ, Liu Y, et al. Biomarkers of rheumatoid arthritis-associated interstitial lung disease. Arthritis Rheum 2015;67(1):28–38.
28. Olson AL, Swigris JJ, Sprunger DB, et al. Rheumatoid arthritis-interstitial lung disease-associated mortality. Am J Respir Crit Care Med 2011;183(3):372–8.
29. Bongartz T, Nannini C, Medina-Velasquez YF, et al. Incidence and mortality of interstitial lung disease in rheumatoid arthritis: a population-based study. Arthritis Rheum 2010;62(6):1583–91.

30. Solomon JJ, Ryu JH, Tazelaar HD, et al. Fibrosing interstitial pneumonia predicts survival in patients with rheumatoid arthritis-associated interstitial lung disease (RA-ILD). Respir Med 2013;107(8):1247–52.

31. Assayag D, Lubin M, Lee JS, et al. Predictors of mortality in rheumatoid arthritis-related interstitial lung disease. Respirology 2014;19(4):493–500.

32. Park JH, Kim DS, Park IN, et al. Prognosis of fibrotic interstitial pneumonia: idiopathic versus collagen vascular disease-related subtypes. Am J Respir Crit Care Med 2007;175(7):705–11.

33. Perez T, Remy-Jardin M, Cortet B. Airways involvement in rheumatoid arthritis: clinical, functional, and HRCT findings. Am J Respir Crit Care Med 1998;157(5 Pt 1):1658–65 [Key Reference].

34. Fischer A, Brown KK, Du Bois RM, et al. Mycophenolate mofetil improves lung function in connective tissue disease-associated interstitial lung disease. J Rheumatol 2013;40(5):640–6.

35. Swigris JJ, Olson AL, Fischer A, et al. Mycophenolate mofetil is safe, well tolerated, and preserves lung function in patients with connective tissue disease-related interstitial lung disease. Chest 2006;130(1):30–6.

36. Keir GJ, Maher TM, Ming D, et al. Rituximab in severe, treatment-refractory interstitial lung disease. Respirology 2014;19(3):353–9.

37. Braun-Moscovici Y, Butbul-Aviel Y, Guralnik L, et al. Rituximab: rescue therapy in life-threatening complications or refractory autoimmune diseases: a single center experience. Rheumatol Int 2013;33(6):1495–504.

38. Chang HK, Park W, Ryu DS. Successful treatment of progressive rheumatoid interstitial lung disease with cyclosporine: a case report. J Korean Med Sci 2002;17(2):270–3 [Key Reference].

39. Puttick MP, Klinkhoff AV, Chalmers A, et al. Treatment of progressive rheumatoid interstitial lung disease with cyclosporine. J Rheumatol 1995;22(11):2163–5.

40. Bargagli E, Galeazzi M, Rottoli P. Infliximab treatment in a patient with rheumatoid arthritis and pulmonary fibrosis. Eur Respir J 2004;24(4):708.

41. Vassallo R, Matteson E, Thomas CF Jr. Clinical response of rheumatoid arthritis-associated pulmonary fibrosis to tumor necrosis factor-alpha inhibition. Chest 2002;122(3):1093–6.

42. Lindsay K, Melsom R, Jacob BK, et al. Acute progression of interstitial lung disease: a complication of etanercept particularly in the presence of rheumatoid lung and methotrexate treatment. Rheumatology (Oxford) 2006;45(8):1048–9.

43. Ostor AJ, Crisp AJ, Somerville MF, et al. Fatal exacerbation of rheumatoid arthritis associated fibrosing alveolitis in patients given infliximab. BMJ 2004;329(7477):1266.

44. Dixon WG, Hyrich KL, Watson KD, et al. Influence of anti-TNF therapy on mortality in patients with rheumatoid arthritis-associated interstitial lung disease: results from the British Society for Rheumatology Biologics Register. Ann Rheum Dis 2010;69(6):1086–91.

45. Yazdani A, Singer LG, Strand V, et al. Survival and quality of life in rheumatoid arthritis-associated interstitial lung disease after lung transplantation. J Heart Lung Transplant 2014;33(5):514–20.

46. Geddes DM, Webley M, Emerson PA. Airways obstruction in rheumatoid arthritis. Ann Rheum Dis 1979;38(3):222–5.

47. Collins RL, Turner RA, Johnson AM, et al. Obstructive pulmonary disease in rheumatoid arthritis. Arthritis Rheum 1976;19(3):623–8.

48. Hassan WU, Keaney NP, Holland CD, et al. Bronchial reactivity and airflow obstruction in rheumatoid arthritis. Ann Rheum Dis 1994;53(8):511–4.

49. Brazeau-Lamontagne L, Charlin B, Levesque RY, et al. Cricoarytenoiditis: CT assessment in rheumatoid arthritis. Radiology 1986;158(2):463–6.
50. Metafratzi ZM, Georgiadis AN, Ioannidou CV, et al. Pulmonary involvement in patients with early rheumatoid arthritis. Scand J Rheumatol 2007;36(5):338–44.
51. Kochbati S, Boussema F, Ben Miled M, et al. Bronchiectasis in rheumatoid arthritis. High resolution computed pulmonary tomography. Tunis Med 2003; 81(10):768–73 [in French].
52. Geri G, Dadoun S, Bui T, et al. Risk of infections in bronchiectasis during disease-modifying treatment and biologics for rheumatic diseases. BMC Infect Dis 2011; 11:304.
53. Pipavath SJ, Lynch DA, Cool C, et al. Radiologic and pathologic features of bronchiolitis. AJR Am J Roentgenol 2005;185(2):354–63.
54. Fernandez Perez ER, Krishnamoorthy M, Brown KK, et al. FEV1 over time in patients with connective tissue disease-related bronchiolitis. Respir Med 2013; 107(6):883–9.
55. Devouassoux G, Cottin V, Liote H, et al. Characterisation of severe obliterative bronchiolitis in rheumatoid arthritis. Eur Respir J 2009;33(5):1053–61.
56. Anaya JM, Diethelm L, Ortiz LA, et al. Pulmonary involvement in rheumatoid arthritis. Semin Arthritis Rheum 1995;24(4):242–54.
57. Walters MN, Ojeda VJ. Pleuropulmonary necrobiotic rheumatoid nodules. A review and clinicopathological study of six patients. Med J Aust 1986;144(12):648–51.
58. Morikawa J, Kitamura K, Habuchi Y, et al. Pulmonary hypertension in a patient with rheumatoid arthritis. Chest 1988;93(4):876–8.
59. Voskuyl AE, Hazes JM, Zwinderman AH, et al. Diagnostic strategy for the assessment of rheumatoid vasculitis. Ann Rheum Dis 2003;62(5):407–13.
60. Avnon LS, Abu-Shakra M, Flusser D, et al. Pleural effusion associated with rheumatoid arthritis: what cell predominance to anticipate? Rheumatol Int 2007; 27(10):919–25.
61. Naylor B. The pathognomonic cytologic picture of rheumatoid pleuritis. The 1989 Maurice Goldblatt Cytology award lecture. Acta Cytol 1990;34(4):465–73.
62. Kremer JM, Alarcon GS, Weinblatt ME, et al. Clinical, laboratory, radiographic, and histopathologic features of methotrexate-associated lung injury in patients with rheumatoid arthritis: a multicenter study with literature review. Arthritis Rheum 1997;40(10):1829–37.
63. Walden PA, Mitchell-Weggs PF, Coppin C, et al. Pleurisy and methotrexate treatment. Br Med J 1977;2(6091):867.
64. Cannon GW, Ward JR, Clegg DO, et al. Acute lung disease associated with low-dose pulse methotrexate therapy in patients with rheumatoid arthritis. Arthritis Rheum 1983;26(10):1269–74.
65. St Clair EW, Rice JR, Snyderman R. Pneumonitis complicating low-dose methotrexate therapy in rheumatoid arthritis. Arch Intern Med 1985;145(11):2035–8.
66. Gispen JG, Alarcon GS, Johnson JJ, et al. Toxicity of methotrexate in rheumatoid arthritis. J Rheumatol 1987;14(1):74–9.
67. Amital A, Shitrit D, Adir Y. The lung in rheumatoid arthritis. Presse Med 2011;40(1 Pt 2):e31–48.
68. Barrera P, Laan RF, van Riel PL, et al. Methotrexate-related pulmonary complications in rheumatoid arthritis. Ann Rheum Dis 1994;53(7):434–9.
69. Toussirot E, Berthelot JM, Pertuiset E, et al. Pulmonary nodulosis and aseptic granulomatous lung disease occurring in patients with rheumatoid arthritis receiving tumor necrosis factor-alpha-blocking agent: a case series. J Rheumatol 2009;36(11):2421–7.

70. Peno-Green L, Lluberas G, Kingsley T, et al. Lung injury linked to etanercept therapy. Chest 2002;122(5):1858–60.

71. Dubey S, Kerrigan N, Mills K, et al. Bronchospasm associated with anti-TNF treatment. Clin Rheumatol 2009;28(8):989–92.

72. Atzeni F, Boiardi L, Salli S, et al. Lung involvement and drug-induced lung disease in patients with rheumatoid arthritis. Expert Rev Clin Immunol 2013;9(7): 649–57.

73. Roubille C, Haraoui B. Interstitial lung diseases induced or exacerbated by DMARDS and biologic agents in rheumatoid arthritis: a systematic literature review. Semin Arthritis Rheum 2014;43(5):613–26.

74. Sakai F, Noma S, Kurihara Y, et al. Leflunomide-related lung injury in patients with rheumatoid arthritis: imaging features. Mod Rheumatol 2005;15(3):173–9.

75. Suissa S, Hudson M, Ernst P. Leflunomide use and the risk of interstitial lung disease in rheumatoid arthritis. Arthritis Rheum 2006;54(5):1435–9.

76. Liote H, Liote F, Seroussi B, et al. Rituximab-induced lung disease: a systematic literature review. Eur Respir J 2010;35(3):681–7.

77. Parry SD, Barbatzas C, Peel ET, et al. Sulphasalazine and lung toxicity. Eur Respir J 2002;19(4):756–64.

78. Hamadeh MA, Atkinson J, Smith LJ. Sulfasalazine-induced pulmonary disease. Chest 1992;101(4):1033–7.

79. Ikegawa K, Hanaoka M, Ushiki A, et al. A case of organizing pneumonia induced by tocilizumab. Intern Med 2011;50(19):2191–3.

80. Kawashiri SY, Kawakami A, Sakamoto N, et al. A fatal case of acute exacerbation of interstitial lung disease in a patient with rheumatoid arthritis during treatment with tocilizumab. Rheumatol Int 2012;32(12):4023–6.

81. Nishimoto N, Yoshizaki K, Miyasaka N, et al. Treatment of rheumatoid arthritis with humanized anti-interleukin-6 receptor antibody: a multicenter, double-blind, placebo-controlled trial. Arthritis Rheum 2004;50(6):1761–9.

# Interstitial Lung Disease in Scleroderma

Sara R. Schoenfeld, MD, Flavia V. Castelino, MD*

## KEYWORDS

- Systemic sclerosis • Interstitial lung disease • Fibrosis • Pathogenesis • Diagnosis
- Treatment

## KEY POINTS

- Interstitial lung disease is a significant cause of morbidity and mortality in systemic sclerosis.
- Diagnostic modalities to assess interstitial lung disease include pulmonary function tests, which may show decreases in the forced vital capacity and diffusion capacity of the lung for carbon monoxide, and high-resolution computed tomography, which may show patterns consistent with nonspecific interstitial pneumonia or usual interstitial pneumonia.
- Pathogenesis revolves around an interplay of vascular injury, inflammation, and subsequent fibrosis, with transforming growth factor-beta playing a key role in fibrosis.
- Effective treatment modalities are limited, with cyclophosphamide being the most rigorously studied treatment. Therapies that are often used in other autoimmune conditions are not as effective in systemic sclerosis-interstitial lung disease.
- Several alternative treatment approaches are being considered, including rituximab, bosentan, tyrosine kinase inhibitors, pirfenidone, and hematopoietic stem cell transplant.

## INTRODUCTION

Systemic sclerosis (SSc) is a heterogeneous disease characterized by vasculopathy, autoimmunity, and fibrosis, with multiorgan involvement and no known cure. Pulmonary complications of SSc remain one of the largest causes of morbidity and mortality in the disease. Interstitial lung disease (ILD) and pulmonary arterial hypertension (PAH) are the most common forms of lung disease associated with SSc. This review focuses on SSc-ILD, a leading cause of mortality in SSc. Pulmonary function tests (PFTs) and chest imaging with high-resolution chest tomography (HRCT) remain important tools

Disclosures: None.
Division of Rheumatology, Massachusetts General Hospital, 55 Fruit Street, Boston, MA 02114, USA
* Corresponding author. Division of Rheumatology, Massachusetts General Hospital, 55 Fruit Street, Yawkey 2C-2100, Boston, MA 02114.
E-mail address: fcastelino@mgh.harvard.edu

Rheum Dis Clin N Am 41 (2015) 237–248
http://dx.doi.org/10.1016/j.rdc.2014.12.005          rheumatic.theclinics.com

in the diagnosis and prognosis of SSc-ILD. Although significant advances have been made in the understanding of the pathogenesis of SSc-ILD, current treatment options have limitations in their overall effectiveness. Several treatment modalities are currently under investigation, and novel targeted treatments that have shown promise in idiopathic pulmonary fibrosis (IPF) clinical trials may ultimately be useful in SSc. This review provides a brief overview of SSc-ILD pathogenesis to date, and includes a discussion of key points in the evaluation and management of the disease, including a discussion on novel therapies.

## EPIDEMIOLOGY

ILD is common in patients with SSc, with up to 90% of patients exhibiting evidence of interstitial changes on HRCT,[1] and between 40% and 75% of patients having PFT abnormalities.[2,3] Clinically significant lung fibrosis is present in approximately 25% of all SSc patients,[4] but there is significant heterogeneity with regard to the incidence of pulmonary involvement based on several factors, including the SSc subset and antibody profile. In particular, patients with diffuse cutaneous SSc (dcSSc) or Scl-70 (anti-topoisomerase) antibodies are at higher risk for ILD development, whereas patients with limited cutaneous SSc or anticentromere antibodies less commonly have ILD. Among 3656 patients in the European League Against Rheumatism (EULAR) Scleroderma Trials and Research database, 60% of patients with positive Scl-70 antibodies had evidence of ILD compared with 21% of patients with anticentromere antibodies.[5] Certain clinical features, such as African-American ethnicity, modified Rodnan Skin Score (mRSS), serum creatinine level, creatine phosphokinase values, and evidence of cardiac involvement are also found to be independent predictors of lung involvement in SSc.[4] In a recent meta-analysis looking at predictors of mortality and progression in SSc-ILD, factors including older age, lower forced vital capacity (FVC), and lower diffusing capacity of the lungs for carbon monoxide (DLCO) predicted mortality.[6] Extent of disease involvement on HRCT predicted both mortality and ILD progression.

Several biomarkers have been studied as possible predictors of the development and progression of ILD in SSc. These markers, which are currently not available for clinical use in the United States, may play a role in prognosis and disease monitoring in the future. Specifically, the glycoproteins Krebs von den Lungen-6 (KL-6) and surfactant protein D (SP-D) are found to be elevated in patients with SSc-ILD, and levels may correlate with ILD severity and progression.[7,8]

## PATHOGENESIS

The pathogenesis of SSc-ILD is multifactorial and incompletely understood. Endothelial cell injury with subsequent vascular damage and alveolar epithelial cell injury are key initial insults that precede fibrosis. At the time of injury, various mediators are released, and fibroblasts are activated. Over time, fibroblasts acquire features of smooth muscle cells and become myofibroblasts, resulting in dysregulated accumulation of collagen and extracellular matrix components and ultimately fibrosis (**Fig. 1**). Some of the mediators implicated in SSc-ILD include thrombin, transforming growth factor-beta (TGF-β), and the Wnt/β-catenin pathway.

### Thrombin

Lung biopsies of SSc-ILD patients show evidence of endothelial and epithelial injury with interstitial edema.[9,10] Endothelial cell injury results in thrombin production and release of endothelin-1 with elevated levels of thrombin detected in bronchoalveolar lavage fluid of SSc patients compared with healthy controls.[11] Inhibition of thrombin

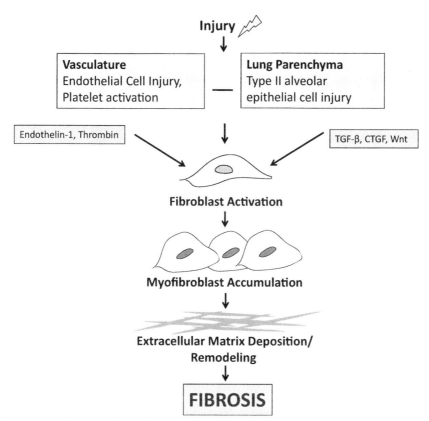

**Fig 1** Key mediators in the pathogenesis of pulmonary fibrosis in SSc. Pulmonary fibrosis is initiated by damage to the vasculature and lung parenchyma, resulting in endothelial and epithelial cell injury. This injury subsequently results in the release of several cytokines and growth factors, which, in turn, activate fibroblasts, resulting in extracellular matrix deposition and ultimately fibrosis. CTGF, connective tissue growth factor.

with the oral direct thrombin inhibitor, dabigatran etexilate (Pradaxa), in the mouse bleomycin model of lung injury reduced the number of inflammatory cells in the bronchoalveolar lavage and decreased lung fibrosis.[12] Both thrombin and endothelin-1 also exert direct effects on fibroblasts and play a role in stimulating TGF-β production, a central mediator of SSc fibrosis.

### Transforming Growth Factor-beta

TGF-β is a pleiotropic cytokine with a central role in SSc-ILD. Once activated, TGF-β binds to its receptor and leads to the phosphorylation of Smad, a group of intracellular signaling proteins.[13,14] The Smad proteins subsequently translocate to the nucleus and act as transcription activators for several genes, including type I collagen, fibronectin, plasminogen activator inhibitor-1, and connective tissue growth factor.[15,16] In mouse models, the conditional knockout of TGF-β receptor type II and Smad3-deficient mice are protected from bleomycin-induced pulmonary fibrosis.[17,18] Trials of small molecule blockade of Smad phosphorylation and of inhibitors of signaling molecules downstream of TGF-β are currently underway and may provide novel targets to treat SSc-ILD.

## Wnt/β-catenin

The Wnt/β-catenin pathway comprises highly conserved growth factors the downstream activity of which leads to the accumulation of β-catenin in the cytoplasm; this then translocates to the nucleus to regulate several genes.[19] Wnt signaling is found to be important in the development of dermal fibrogenesis and the suppression of adipogenesis in a mouse model and in SSc patients.[20,21] In addition, aberrant expression of components of the Wnt/β-catenin pathway has been implicated in the pathogenesis of IPF.[22,23] Administration of an antibody to the downstream molecule Wnt1-inducible signaling protein-1 was associated with a decrease in collagen and improved lung function in a mouse model,[23] and further exploration into blockade of the Wnt/β-catenin pathway may provide additional therapeutic strategies for patients with SSc-ILD.

## CLINICAL MANIFESTATIONS

Patients with mild ILD may be asymptomatic during the early stages of the disease. As the extent of pulmonary fibrosis increases, patients often report fatigue and dyspnea on exertion, and physical examination may find dry "velcro" crackles at the lung bases. Of note, patients with PAH may also have exertional dyspnea and fatigue, and the clinician must keep both entities in mind when evaluating an SSc patient for dyspnea. Dry cough is often present and may correlate with DLCO and dyspnea.[24] In the Scleroderma Lung Study, cough severity improved in patients treated with cyclophosphamide, but these improvements disappeared after 2 years of follow-up.[25,26]

## IMAGING FINDINGS

HRCT plays an important role in determining the pattern and extent of involvement of ILD in SSc patients. The most common pattern seen on HRCT is nonspecific interstitial pneumonia (NSIP), although usual interstitial pneumonia (UIP) can also be seen in 25% to 40% of cases.[25,27] The NSIP pattern on HRCT is evident by ground glass opacities in a peripheral distribution with subpleural and basilar predominance (**Fig. 2**A). In more severe disease, volume loss with a reticular pattern and traction bronchiectasis can also be seen. In UIP, HRCT findings include reticulonodular opacities, traction bronchiectasis, and honeycomb cysts (see **Fig. 2**B). A normal chest computed tomography

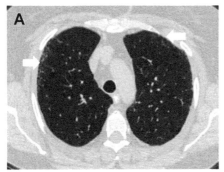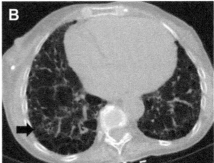

**Fig. 2.** Representative radiographic findings on high-resolution computed tomography. (*A*) Subpleural ground glass opacities (*white arrows*) and traction bronchiectasis consistent with nonspecific interstitial pneumonia, and (*B*) Honeycombing (*black arrow*), bronchiectasis, and ground glass opacities suggestive of usual interstitial pneumonia.

scan at baseline is generally reassuring; in one study, 85% of SSc patients who had a normal HRCT at baseline still had a normal HRCT at 5 years.[28]

## PULMONARY FUNCTION TESTS

PFTs are a key component in the diagnosis and long-term follow-up of SSc-ILD. The FVC and DLCO are important parameters for the assessment of lung function in SSc patients, and the FVC can help stratify patients for treatment.[29] Reduced DLCO is sensitive for early ILD but can also be an indicator of pulmonary hypertension and needs to be interpreted in the context of the overall lung volumes. FVC and DLCO should be greater than 80% predicted to be considered normal. In a study of 890 SSc patients who had PFTs, 60% had no or minimal restrictive disease (FVC >75%), 27% had moderate disease (FVC 50%–75%), and 14% had severe disease (FVC ≤50%).[3] Both FVC and DLCO are prognostic factors in patients with SSc-ILD. Among 80 patients who underwent lung biopsy for SSc with fibrosing alveolitis, lower initial DLCO and FVC were associated with mortality.[27]

In general, the authors recommend close clinical follow-up of SSc patients to monitor for a change in cardiopulmonary symptoms, usually every 3 to 6 months. In the absence of a clinical change, PFTs should be done annually. If there is progression of symptoms, such as dyspnea or cough, PFTs should be done every 6 months and should be followed with an HRCT if there are abnormalities on the PFTs. Others have suggested that HRCT be performed in all SSc patients as a screening examination and, if mildly abnormal, be followed by PFTs every 3 to 6 months.[30] Both HRCT and PFTs are well-accepted methods for the diagnosis of SSc-ILD, with 100% and 99% consensus among 117 SSc experts for the use of HRCT and PFTs, respectively.[31] The first 5 years after diagnosis of SSc are critical for the development of ILD, and patients should be monitored closely during this time. The clinician should also keep in mind the role that gastroesophageal reflux (GER) may play in worsening fibrosis and clinical symptoms.[32] Patients with SSc-ILD are found to have more severe GER than SSc patients without ILD,[33] and this may contribute to worsening respiratory symptoms.

## 6-MINUTE WALK TEST

The 6-minute walk test (6MWT) is an easy and noninvasive tool used for the assessment of lung function in pulmonary disease. Its utility in SSc-ILD is, however, limited primarily because of functional impairment of patients. In a study of 163 patients with SSc-ILD, the 6MWT did not correlate well with other parameters such as FVC, DLCO, or dyspnea index scores despite its reproducibility.[34] It may play a more important role in SSc patients with PAH.

## HISTOPATHOLOGY

Histologically, SSc-ILD is characterized by early pulmonary infiltration of inflammatory cells and subsequent fibrosis of the lung parenchyma. The most common patterns seen on histologic examination are NSIP and UIP. NSIP is characterized by varying degrees of inflammation and fibrosis. In contrast, UIP is characterized by dense patchy fibrosis with "honeycombing," primarily in a subpleural distribution. NSIP is the more common pattern seen in SSc-ILD and is present in 64% to 77% of cases.[27,35] Lung biopsy is not necessary to confirm the histopathologic diagnosis, as the patterns of ILD are usually readily distinguishable on HRCT. Biopsy may play a role when other diagnoses, such as infection or malignancy, are suspected based on HRCT.

## TREATMENT
### Approach to Treatment

Multiple treatment modalities have been used in SSc-ILD with only some having modest benefit. Drug development for ILD has expanded dramatically and several investigational approaches are currently in early-phase clinical trials. The decision of which patients to treat must be considered carefully given the potential toxicities of many of the medications. An algorithm for determining the severity of disease has been proposed by Goh and colleagues,[29] and use of this algorithm may aid in treatment decisions for a patient with SSc-ILD. In this algorithm, lung involvement on HRCT of greater than 20% and FVC less than 70% were associated with increased mortality risk, and these parameters may help determine which patients would benefit the most from treatment.

### Current Treatment Modalities

#### Cyclophosphamide (Cytoxan)

Cyclophosphamide (Cytoxan) has been the most rigorously studied medication in the treatment of SSc-ILD (**Table 1**). The 2009 EULAR recommendations for the treatment of SSc suggest the use of cyclophosphamide for the treatment of SSc-ILD despite its known potential toxicities.[36] This recommendation was based on 2 randomized, controlled trials (RCTs) comparing cyclophosphamide with placebo. In a small study of patients with SSc-ILD, monthly intravenous cyclophosphamide for 6 months, in addition to prednisolone followed by azathioprine, was compared with placebo.[37] There was a trend toward improvement in FVC, but this did not reach statistical significance likely in part because of the small study size. In the first multicenter RCT to look at the role of cyclophosphamide in SSc-ILD, the Scleroderma Lung Study found that patients with early SSc-ILD treated with oral cyclophosphamide for 1 year had improvement in FVC, dyspnea index scores, chest imaging, and skin scores, but not in DLCO.[25] By 2 years, the positive effect of cyclophosphamide on lung function had disappeared, but the improvement in dyspnea scores was still present.[26] Based on these results, cyclophosphamide should be strongly considered as first-line treatment in patients with SSc-ILD. The optimal duration of therapy is not known given the

| Table 1 Current treatment options for SSc-ILD | | |
|---|---|---|
| **Drug** | **Mechanism of Action** | **Data Supporting Use** |
| Cyclophosphamide | Alkylating agent, cross-links DNA, decreasing DNA synthesis and preventing cell division | Scleroderma Lung Study (multicenter RCT), improvement in FVC, dyspnea scores, chest imaging[25] |
| Mycophenolate mofetil | Inhibits inosine monophosphate dehydrogenase, inhibits de novo guanosine nucleotide synthesis, prevents T and B proliferation | Observational studies, stabilization or improvement in FVC or DLCO[39–41] Scleroderma Lung Study II ongoing |
| Azathioprine | Metabolites incorporated into replicating DNA, blocks the pathway for purine synthesis | Observational studies, both alone and after cyclophosphamide, stabilization or improvement in FVC and dyspnea scores.[37,43,44] |
| Lung transplant | Not applicable | Similar survival rates as non–SSc-ILD patients[45,46] |

risk of adverse effects; typical protocols suggest treatment up to a year followed by a switch to another agent for maintenance therapy (see later discussion).[38]

### Mycophenolate mofetil (Cellcept)

Several retrospective and case-control studies suggest that mycophenolate mofetil (MMF; Cellcept) may have a beneficial effect on SSc-ILD. In these studies, treatment with MMF resulted in stabilization or improvement of either FVC or DCLO during the treatment period, whereas lung function had declined in the period preceding treatment with MMF.[39–41] However, a retrospective case-control study that compared patients with SSc-ILD treated with MMF versus cyclophosphamide versus control found that PFTs and clinical parameters were similar but that radiographic findings on HRCT worsened in the group treated with MMF despite being a less sick group at onset.[42] The Scleroderma Lung Study II, which is currently ongoing, will compare 1 year of oral cyclophosphamide with 2 years of MMF for the treatment of SSc-ILD and should provide further information on the utility of MMF in SSc-ILD (ClinicalTrials.gov Identifier: NCT00883129). MMF may provide a good option for maintenance therapy for patients with SSc-ILD after induction with cyclophosphamide.[31]

### Azathioprine (Imuran)

Azathioprine (Imuran) may have a role as an alternative agent to cyclophosphamide or as a maintenance medication after initial treatment with cyclophosphamide. In a retrospective study of 11 patients with SSc-ILD, treatment with azathioprine resulted in stable FVC and dyspnea index scores in 8 patients.[43] In another study of SSc-ILD patients with worsening lung function, treatment with 6 months of monthly intravenous cyclophosphamide followed by 18 months of azathioprine resulted in stable or improved PFTs at 6 months in 70% of patients.[44]

### Role of lung transplant

Lung transplant remains an option for patients who do not respond to conventional medical management. There are concerns about whether involvement of other organ systems may pose a problem in the overall prognosis of SSc patients who undergo transplant, specifically whether patients with severe GER may have recurrent aspiration events leading to increased lung damage. However, studies comparing outcomes after lung transplant in SSc-ILD patients with those of other ILD patients show similar 1- and 5-year survival rates.[45,46]

### Investigational Approaches

### Rituximab (Rituxan)

Results of several trials show potentially promising results supporting the use of rituximab (Rituxan) in SSc-ILD (**Table 2**). A recent study found that SSc patients treated with rituximab had a greater improvement in skin score and had less decline in FVC compared with controls.[47] A smaller study of 14 patients with SSc-ILD treated with rituximab showed similar improvements in lung function and skin scores.[48] Further multicenter randomized studies are needed to determine whether rituximab may be a reasonable alternative to cyclophosphamide as a first-line treatment for SSc-ILD.

### Bosentan (Tracleer)

Bosentan (Tracleer) is an endothelin-1 antagonist that is frequently used in SSc-associated PAH and has been investigated in SSc-ILD. The Bosentan in Interstitial Lung Disease in Systemic Sclerosis-2 (BUILD-2) study randomly assigned patients with SSc-ILD to bosentan or placebo and found no difference in the 6MWT or in PFTs between the 2 groups at 12 months.[49] Of note, the BUILD-3 trial evaluating

**Table 2**
**Investigational treatments for SSc-ILD**

| Drug | Mechanism of Action | Data Supporting Use |
|------|--------------------|--------------------|
| Rituximab | Monoclonal antibody against CD20 on B-lymphocytes | Small randomized trials, less decline or improvement in FVC[47,48] |
| Bosentan | Endothelin-1 receptor antagonist | BUILD-2 (RCT), no difference in PFTs or 6MWT[49] |
| Imatinib | Tyrosine kinase inhibitor | Open-label trials, one with improvement in FVC, one with no change in DLCO[51,52] |
| Pirfenidone | Antifibrotic and anti-inflammatory effects | ASCEND (RCT in IPF), improvement in FVC and progression-free survival in IPF[54] LOTUSS, ongoing |
| HSCT | Lymphocyte ablation | ASSIST, improvement in FVC[55] ASTIS, improved event-free and overall survival[56] SCOT, ongoing |

bosentan in IPF failed to reach its primary endpoints of time to worsening IPF or death.[50]

*Tyrosine kinase inhibitors*
Studies of tyrosine kinase inhibitors such as imatinib (Gleevec) in SSc-ILD have had variable results. In one open-label, phase II trial, 30 patients with diffuse SSc were treated with imatinib for 12 months.[51] Overall, there was improvement in both the mRSS and FVC, although only half of the patients had ILD at baseline. Another study treated 28 patients with morphea or diffuse SSc with 6 months of either imatinib or placebo and found no difference in the change in mRSS or DLCO between the 2 groups.[52] A larger RCT of imatinib versus placebo in IPF patients did not show any effect on lung function or survival.[53]

*Pirfenidone (Esbriet)*
Pirfenidone (Esbriet) has been studied extensively in IPF and has both anti-inflammatory and antifibrotic effects. A recent large multicenter RCT of pirfenidone in IPF patients found less disease progression, as measured by FVC, improved progression-free survival, and reduced decline in the 6MWT in patients receiving pirfenidone.[54] Pirfenidone has been granted breakthrough therapy designation from the US Food and Drug Administration for use in IPF. A phase II study of pirfenidone in SSc-ILD is currently underway (LOTUSS Study, ClinicalTrials.gov Identifier: NCT01933334).

*Autologous stem cell transplant*
Autologous hematopoietic stem cell transplant (HSCT) has been studied as an attractive alternative therapeutic option given the poor prognosis of patients with SSc-ILD. Three major trials, one still ongoing, compared HSCT with cyclophosphamide in SSc patients with internal organ involvement. The ASSIST (Autologous Stem Cell Systemic Sclerosis Immune Suppression Trial) study randomly assigned 19 patients with dcSSc and internal organ or pulmonary involvement to either nonmyeloablative autologous HSCT or monthly intravenous cyclophosphamide for 6 months.[55] All patients in the HSCT group had improved skin scores and FVC at 12 months compared with none in the cyclophosphamide group, and 7 of 9 patients in the cyclophosphamide group were switched to the HSCT group. The ASTIS (Autologous Stem cell Transplantation International Scleroderma) trial compared HSCT with 12 months of monthly

intravenous cyclophosphamide in 156 patients with dcSSc; patients in the HSCT group had improved event-free and overall survival despite a 10% treatment-related mortality rate in the HSCT group.[56] The SCOT (Scleroderma: Cyclophosphamide Or Transplantation) trial is currently ongoing (ClinicalTrials.gov Identifier: NCT00114530). HSCT may be an option for patients with severe disease who have been refractory to other treatment options.

## PROGNOSIS

The overall prognosis of SSc-ILD is poor, but there is variability between the different pathologic subsets. Patients with NSIP tend to have better outcomes, with a median survival of 15 years compared with 3 years in patients with UIP.[27] Factors such as older age, lower FVC, and lower DLCO are predictive of mortality in SSc-ILD, and extent of disease on HRCT often predicts mortality and ILD progression.[6] Particular attention should be paid to these parameters when evaluating patients with SSc-ILD.

## SUMMARY

ILD is one of the most serious complications among patients with SSc, and despite advances in the understanding of the pathogenesis and treatment of the disease there is still significant morbidity and mortality. PFTs and HRCT play a central role in the diagnosis of ILD and should be monitored routinely. Although certain subgroups of SSc patients seem to be at higher risk for ILD development, we do not have clear biomarkers for which patients will get the disease or have disease progression. Treatment modalities that are often used with success in other autoimmune diseases have proven less beneficial in SSc-ILD. Cyclophosphamide remains the best-studied agent and should be considered for any patient with progressive SSc-ILD. Newer investigational treatments such as rituximab, pirfenidone, and HSCT may become options as further studies shed light on their potential benefit. Further understanding of the pathogenesis and molecular mediators will ultimately lead to novel treatment targets to modify the course of SSc-ILD.

## REFERENCES

1. Churawitzki H, Stiglbauer R, Graninger W, et al. Interstitial lung disease in progressive systemic sclerosis: high-resolution CT versus radiography. Radiology 1990;176(3):755–9.
2. Steen VD, Owens GR, Fino GJ, et al. Pulmonary involvement in systemic sclerosis (scleroderma). Arthritis Rheum 1985;28(7):759–67.
3. Steen VD, Conte C, Owens GR, et al. Severe restrictive lung disease in systemic sclerosis. Arthritis Rheum 1994;37(9):1283–9.
4. McNearney TA, Reveille JD, Fischbach M, et al. Pulmonary involvement in systemic sclerosis: associations with genetic, serologic, sociodemographic, and behavioral factors. Arthritis Rheum 2007;57(2):318–26.
5. Walker UA, Tyndall A, Czirjak L, et al. Clinical risk assessment of organ manifestations in systemic sclerosis: a report from the EULAR scleroderma trials and research group database. Ann Rheum Dis 2007;66(6):754–63.
6. Winstone TA, Assayag D, Wilcox PG, et al. Predictors of mortality and progression in scleroderma-associated interstitial lung disease: a systematic review. Chest 2014;146(2):422–36.

7. Yanaba K, Hasegawa M, Hamaguchi Y, et al. Longitudinal analysis of serum KL-6 levels in patients with systemic sclerosis: association with the activity of pulmonary fibrosis. Clin Exp Rheumatol 2003;21(4):429–36.

8. Yanaba K, Hasegawa M, Takehara K, et al. Comparative study of serum surfactant protein-D and KL-6 concentrations in patients with systemic sclerosis as markers for monitoring the activity of pulmonary fibrosis. J Rheumatol 2004;31(6):1112–20.

9. Harrison NK, Myers AR, Corrin B, et al. Structural features of interstitial lung disease in systemic sclerosis. Am Rev Respir Dis 1991;144(3 Pt 1):706–13.

10. Jain S, Shahane A, Derk CT. Interstitial lung disease in systemic sclerosis: pathophysiology, current and new advances in therapy. Inflamm Allergy Drug Targets 2012;11(4):266–77.

11. Ohba T, McDonald JK, Silver RM, et al. Scleroderma bronchoalveolar lavage fluid contains thrombin, a mediator of human lung fibroblast proliferation via induction of platelet-derived growth factor alpha-receptor. Am J Respir Cell Mol Biol 1994;10(4):405–12.

12. Bogatkevich GS, Ludwicka-Bradley A, Nietert PJ, et al. Antiinflammatory and antifibrotic effects of the oral direct thrombin inhibitor dabigatran etexilate in a murine model of interstitial lung disease. Arthritis Rheum 2011;63(5):1416–25.

13. Akter T, Silver RM, Bogatkevich GS. Recent advances in understanding the pathogenesis of scleroderma-interstitial lung disease. Curr Rheumatol Rep 2014;16(4):411.

14. Mauviel A. Transforming growth factor-beta: a key mediator of fibrosis. Methods Mol Med 2005;117:69–80.

15. Willis BC, Borok Z. TGF-beta-induced EMT: mechanisms and implications for fibrotic lung disease. Am J Physiol Lung Cell Mol Physiol 2007;293(3):L525–34.

16. Varga J, Abraham D. Systemic sclerosis: a prototypic multisystem fibrotic disorder. J Clin Invest 2007;117(3):557–67.

17. Li M, Krishnaveni MS, Li C, et al. Epithelium-specific deletion of TGF-beta receptor type II protects mice from bleomycin-induced pulmonary fibrosis. J Clin Invest 2011;121(1):277–87.

18. Zhao J, Shi W, Wang YL, et al. Smad3 deficiency attenuates bleomycin-induced pulmonary fibrosis in mice. Am J Physiol Lung Cell Mol Physiol 2002;282(3):L585–93.

19. Clevers H, Nusse R. WNT/beta-catenin signaling and disease. Cell 2012;149(6):1192–205.

20. Wei J, Melichian D, Komura K, et al. Canonical Wnt signaling induces skin fibrosis and subcutaneous lipoatrophy: a novel mouse model for scleroderma? Arthritis Rheum 2011;63(6):1707–17.

21. Wei J, Fang F, Lam AP, et al. WNT/beta-catenin signaling is hyperactivated in systemic sclerosis and induces Smad-dependent fibrotic responses in mesenchymal cells. Arthritis Rheum 2012;64(8):2734–45.

22. Chilosi M, Poletti V, Zamo A, et al. Aberrant Wnt/beta-catenin pathway activation in idiopathic pulmonary fibrosis. Am J Pathol 2003;162(5):1495–502.

23. Konigshoff M, Kramer M, Balsara N, et al. WNT1-inducible signaling protein-1 mediates pulmonary fibrosis in mice and is upregulated in humans with idiopathic pulmonary fibrosis. J Clin Invest 2009;119(4):772–87.

24. Theodore AC, Tseng CH, Li N, et al. Correlation of cough with disease activity and treatment with cyclophosphamide in scleroderma interstitial lung disease: findings from the Scleroderma Lung Study. Chest 2012;142(3):614–21.

25. Tashkin DP, Elashoff R, Clements PJ, et al. Cyclophosphamide versus placebo in scleroderma lung disease. N Engl J Med 2006;354(25):2655–66.

26. Tashkin DP, Elashoff R, Clements PJ, et al. Effects of 1-year treatment with cyclophosphamide on outcomes at 2 years in scleroderma lung disease. Am J Respir Crit Care Med 2007;176(10):1026–34.

27. Bouros D, Wells AU, Nicholson AG, et al. Histopathologic subsets of fibrosing alveolitis in patients with systemic sclerosis and their relationship to outcome. Am J Respir Crit Care Med 2002;165(12):1581–6.

28. Launay D, Remy-Jardin M, Michon-Pasturel U, et al. High resolution computed tomography in fibrosing alveolitis associated with systemic sclerosis. J Rheumatol 2006;33(9):1789–801.

29. Goh NS, Desai SR, Veeraraghavan S, et al. Interstitial lung disease in systemic sclerosis: a simple staging system. Am J Respir Crit Care Med 2008;177(11):1248–54.

30. Solomon JJ, Olson AL, Fischer A, et al. Scleroderma lung disease. Eur Respir Rev 2013;22(127):6–19.

31. Walker KM, Pope J, Participating members of the Scleroderma Clinical Trials Consortium (SCTC), et al. Treatment of systemic sclerosis complications: what to use when first-line treatment fails–a consensus of systemic sclerosis experts. Semin Arthritis Rheum 2012;42(1):42–55.

32. Christmann RB, Wells AU, Capelozzi VL, et al. Gastroesophageal reflux incites interstitial lung disease in systemic sclerosis: clinical, radiologic, histopathologic, and treatment evidence. Semin Arthritis Rheum 2010;40(3):241–9.

33. Savarino E, Bazzica M, Zentilin P, et al. Gastroesophageal reflux and pulmonary fibrosis in scleroderma: a study using pH-impedance monitoring. Am J Respir Crit Care Med 2009;179(5):408–13.

34. Buch MH, Denton CP, Furst DE, et al. Submaximal exercise testing in the assessment of interstitial lung disease secondary to systemic sclerosis: reproducibility and correlations of the 6-min walk test. Ann Rheum Dis 2007;66(2):169–73.

35. Fischer A, Swigris JJ, Groshong SD, et al. Clinically significant interstitial lung disease in limited scleroderma: histopathology, clinical features, and survival. Chest 2008;134(3):601–5.

36. Kowal-Bielecka O, Landewe R, Avouac J, et al. EULAR recommendations for the treatment of systemic sclerosis: a report from the EULAR Scleroderma Trials and Research group (EUSTAR). Ann Rheum Dis 2009;68(5):620–8.

37. Hoyles RK, Ellis RW, Wellsbury J, et al. A multicenter, prospective, randomized, double-blind, placebo-controlled trial of corticosteroids and intravenous cyclophosphamide followed by oral azathioprine for the treatment of pulmonary fibrosis in scleroderma. Arthritis Rheum 2006;54(12):3962–70.

38. Hoffman GS, Kerr GS, Leavitt RY, et al. Wegener granulomatosis: an analysis of 150 patients. Ann Intern Med 1992;116(6):488–98.

39. Gerbino AJ, Goss CH, Molitor JA. Effect of mycophenolate mofetil on pulmonary function in scleroderma-associated interstitial lung disease. Chest 2008;133(2):455–60.

40. Simeon-Aznar CP, Fonollosa-Pla V, Tolosa-Vilella C, et al. Effect of mycophenolate sodium in scleroderma-related interstitial lung disease. Clin Rheumatol 2011;30(11):1393–8.

41. Zamora AC, Wolters PJ, Collard HR, et al. Use of mycophenolate mofetil to treat scleroderma-associated interstitial lung disease. Respir Med 2008;102(1):150–5.

42. Panopoulos ST, Bournia VK, Trakada G, et al. Mycophenolate versus cyclophosphamide for progressive interstitial lung disease associated with systemic sclerosis: a 2-year case control study. Lung 2013;191(5):483–9.

43. Dheda K, Lalloo UG, Cassim B, et al. Experience with azathioprine in systemic sclerosis associated with interstitial lung disease. Clin Rheumatol 2004;23(4):306–9.

44. Berezne A, Ranque B, Valeyre D, et al. Therapeutic strategy combining intrave-nous cyclophosphamide followed by oral azathioprine to treat worsening interstitial lung disease associated with systemic sclerosis: a retrospective multicenter open-label study. J Rheumatol 2008;35(6):1064–72.

45. Sottile PD, Iturbe D, Katsumoto TR, et al. Outcomes in systemic sclerosis-related lung disease after lung transplantation. Transplantation 2013;95(7):975–80.

46. Schachna L, Medsger TA Jr, Dauber JH, et al. Lung transplantation in sclero-derma compared with idiopathic pulmonary fibrosis and idiopathic pulmonary arterial hypertension. Arthritis Rheum 2006;54(12):3954–61.

47. Jordan S, Distler JH, Maurer B, et al. Effects and safety of rituximab in systemic sclerosis: an analysis from the European Scleroderma Trial and Research (EUSTAR) group. Ann Rheum Dis 2014. [Epub ahead of print].

48. Daoussis D, Liossis SN, Tsamandas AC, et al. Experience with rituximab in scleroderma: results from a 1-year, proof-of-principle study. Rheumatology (Oxford) 2010;49(2):271–80.

49. Seibold JR, Denton CP, Furst DE, et al. Randomized, prospective, placebo-controlled trial of bosentan in interstitial lung disease secondary to systemic scle-rosis. Arthritis Rheum 2010;62(7):2101–8.

50. King TE Jr, Brown KK, Raghu G, et al. BUILD-3: a randomized, controlled trial of bosentan in idiopathic pulmonary fibrosis. Am J Respir Crit Care Med 2011; 184(1):92–9.

51. Khanna D, Saggar R, Mayes MD, et al. A one-year, phase I/IIa, open-label pilot trial of imatinib mesylate in the treatment of systemic sclerosis-associated active interstitial lung disease. Arthritis Rheum 2011;63(11):3540–6.

52. Prey S, Ezzedine K, Doussau A, et al. Imatinib mesylate in scleroderma-associated diffuse skin fibrosis: a phase II multicentre randomized double-blinded controlled trial. Br J Dermatol 2012;167(5):1138–44.

53. Daniels CE, Lasky JA, Limper AH, et al. Imatinib treatment for idiopathic pulmo-nary fibrosis: Randomized placebo-controlled trial results. Am J Respir Crit Care Med 2010;181(6):604–10.

54. King TE Jr, Bradford WZ, Castro-Bernardini S, et al. A phase 3 trial of pirfenidone in patients with idiopathic pulmonary fibrosis. N Engl J Med 2014;370(22): 2083–92.

55. Burt RK, Shah SJ, Dill K, et al. Autologous non-myeloablative haemopoietic stem-cell transplantation compared with pulse cyclophosphamide once per month for systemic sclerosis (ASSIST): an open-label, randomised phase 2 trial. Lancet 2011;378(9790):498–506.

56. van Laar JM, Farge D, Sont JK, et al. Autologous hematopoietic stem cell trans-plantation vs intravenous pulse cyclophosphamide in diffuse cutaneous systemic sclerosis: a randomized clinical trial. JAMA 2014;311(24):2490–8.

# Pulmonary Complications of Inflammatory Myopathy

Shelly A. Miller, MD[a], Marilyn K. Glassberg, MD[a], Dana P. Ascherman, MD[b],*

## KEYWORDS

- Inflammatory myopathy • Polymyositis • Dermatomyositis
- Interstitial lung disease (ILD) • Autoantibodies

## KEY POINTS

- Up to 75% of patients with inflammatory myopathy develop pulmonary involvement in the form of interstitial lung disease (ILD). It is an independent predictor of mortality, and the number 1 cause of disease-related death in idiopathic inflammatory myopathies.
- Secondary pulmonary complications include aspiration pneumonia, opportunistic infections, spontaneous pneumomediastinum, pulmonary hypertension, ventilatory failure caused by neuromuscular weakness, and drug-induced pneumonitis.
- The antisynthetase syndrome is characterized by the presence of anti-ARS (anti–aminoacyl transfer RNA synthetase) antibodies in combination with ILD and/or myositis. Anti–Jo-1 is the most common anti-ARS antibody and is associated with a high risk of ILD.
- Nonspecific interstitial pneumonia is the most common histopathologic diagnosis, but ILD can also be in the form of usual interstitial pneumonia, cryptogenic organizing pneumonia, diffuse alveolar hemorrhage, and acute respiratory distress syndrome.
- Corticosteroids are the mainstay of therapy, but additional immunosuppressive agents are often required.

## INTRODUCTION

The idiopathic inflammatory myopathies (IIMs) are immune-mediated, systemic inflammatory diseases that manifest with varying degrees of muscle inflammation. They primarily include polymyositis (PM), dermatomyositis (DM), and inclusion body myositis (IBM). There are also patients with amyopathic dermatomyositis who present with the hallmark skin findings of DM, but lack significant muscle involvement. The presence of circulating antibodies in the serum of affected patients along with muscle

Disclosures: None.
[a] Division of Pulmonary, Allergy, Critical Care, and Sleep Medicine, University of Miami Miller School of Medicine, 1600 NW 10th Avenue, #1140, Miami, FL 33136, USA; [b] Division of Rheumatology, University of Miami Miller School of Medicine, Rosenstiel Medical Science Building 7152, 1600 Northwest 10th Avenue, Miami, FL 33136-1050, USA
* Corresponding author.
E-mail address: dascherman@med.miami.edu

tissue specimens containing T cells, macrophages, dendritic cells, B-lymphocytes, and plasma cells confirm that these diseases are immune mediated. Illustrating the systemic nature of IIM, these inflammatory processes often extend to other organ systems, most notably the lungs.[1]

There are multiple secondary pulmonary complications associated with the inflammatory myopathies, but a significant number of patients are also affected with an intrinsic form of interstitial lung disease (ILD). Mills and Mathews[2] first described ILD in a patient with dermatomyositis in 1956, and studies now estimate that 21% to 78% of patients with IIM have pulmonary involvement.[3] ILD has not only been associated with a higher morbidity and mortality in this population, but has also proved to be an independent risk factor for death.[4] In fact, pulmonary involvement is the leading cause of disease-related death among patients with IIM[5] and therefore should be prioritized as part of ongoing management and future investigations.

## SECONDARY PULMONARY COMPLICATIONS

Although ILD affects many patients with inflammatory myopathy, there are secondary pulmonary complications to consider as well. These complications include aspiration pneumonitis/pneumonia, spontaneous pneumomediastinum, opportunistic infections, pulmonary hypertension, ventilatory failure caused by muscle weakness, and drug-induced pneumonitis (**Table 1**).

### Aspiration Pneumonitis

Among patients with PM/DM, the lung is the most common site of pyogenic infection, which is usually secondary to aspiration pneumonia.[6] One study found that aspiration pneumonia occurs in up to one-fifth (15%–20%) of patients with PM/DM. Marie and colleagues[6] studied 279 patients with inflammatory myopathy and found that two-thirds of pyogenic infections were related to aspiration pneumonia. One-fourth of these patients also had ILD on their chest imaging, and 17% of these patients died because of pneumonia-related complications within 1 year of PM/DM diagnosis. These findings suggest a high prevalence of aspiration that represents a potentially modifiable risk factor for worsening pulmonary outcomes.

Associated with this problem of aspiration pneumonitis that may be caused by nasopharyngeal dysfunction, studies have proved that patients with ILD have a higher prevalence of abnormal acid exposure in the proximal and distal esophagus compared to those without ILD. Although this problem does not seem to stem (directly) from the proximal esophageal dysfunction that can complicate inflammatory myopathy, it is likely prevalent among patients with IIM. Many of these patients do not have symptoms of gastroesophageal reflux[7]; although it is standard for proton pump

| Table 1 | |
|---|---|
| **Secondary pulmonary complications of IIM** | |
| **Secondary Pulmonary Complication** | **Prevalence in IIM (%)** |
| Aspiration pneumonia/pneumonitis | 15–20[6,7] |
| Opportunistic infection | 11–21[11,69] |
| Pulmonary hypertension | ~8[12] |
| Spontaneous pneumomediastinum | ~8[15] |
| Ventilatory failure caused by neuromuscular weakness | Unknown |
| Drug-induced pneumonitis | Unknown |

inhibitor therapy to be given to help prevent microaspiration, future studies are needed to prove long-term benefit.

### Opportunistic Infections

The treatment of active inflammatory myopathy includes immunosuppressive medications and, as a result, patients undergoing pharmacotherapy are more prone to infection. The opportunistic lung infections are most commonly caused by fungi, which accounted for about 40% of cases in a study conducted by Marie and colleagues[6] in 2011. However, although the guidelines for *Pneumocystis jiroveci* pneumonia (PCP) prophylaxis are clear when it comes to patients with human immunodeficiency virus, they are not as straightforward for other immunosuppressed populations.[8]

Steroids are the first-line therapy for active inflammatory myopathy and are often given in high doses to achieve a clinical response. Enomoto and colleagues[9] conducted a retrospective analysis of 74 patients with idiopathic ILD to assess the incidence of PCP in those patients treated with corticosteroids. All of the patients received more than 0.5 mg/kg of prednisolone with or without additional immunosuppressants for more than 3 weeks. The mean dose of glucocorticoids was 37 mg daily. Seven out of 74 patients developed PCP, but none of those who were taking Bactrim as prophylaxis were affected. Multiple other studies have shown a significant risk of PCP in patients on biologic agents and disease-modifying antirheumatic drugs[10,11] (complementing some of the older literature regarding the risk of PCP in patients with granulomatosis with polyangiitis/Wegener's receiving a combination of corticosteroids and cyclophosphamide), indicating that primary prophylaxis should be considered in this population despite the lack of clear guidelines.

### Congestive Heart Failure

Cardiac muscle tends not to be affected directly by the primary disease process because of inherent differences between cardiac and skeletal muscle. However, many of these patients have significant comorbidities at the time of diagnosis, or develop them during the course of disease. Congestive heart failure should therefore be considered in any patient presenting with dyspnea and bilateral interstitial infiltrates.

### Pulmonary Hypertension

Pulmonary hypertension affects approximately 8% of patients with PM/DM[12] and correlates independently with a lower 3-year survival rate. Although pulmonary hypertension can develop in the later stages of ILD secondary to significant fibrosis and chronic hypoxemia, at least one study showed that ILD was not significantly more prevalent in those with pulmonary hypertension than in those without, suggesting that there may be an intrinsic vascular component.[12] A smaller case series of 20 patients showed that 20% had pulmonary arterial medial and intimal hypertrophy on biopsy, hinting at possible pathogenesis.[13] Despite these considerations, studies have not yet proved any clear benefit to standard pulmonary vasodilator therapy in this patient population; nevertheless, the use of two-dimensional echocardiography to screen for pulmonary hypertension may be of some prognostic value.

### Ventilatory Failure Caused by Muscle Weakness

In severe cases of inflammatory myopathy, patients may have pharyngeal and respiratory muscle weakness, which ultimately result in respiratory failure. Weakness of the respiratory musculature can be objectively assessed through measurement of the maximal inspiratory force (MIF) and maximal expiratory force (MEF). Although corticosteroids and other immunosuppressive agents are the mainstays of treatment of underlying myositis, not all patients respond. Maintenance therapy with noninvasive positive pressure ventilation improves quality of life, and, in severe cases, tracheostomy with home mechanical ventilation can be lifesaving.[14]

### Spontaneous Pneumomediastinum

Spontaneous pneumomediastinum is a rare complication of ILD that can result in free air around mediastinal structures. One study estimated its prevalence to be approximately 8.3% among patients with PM/DM, which is the most frequent connective tissue disease with which it is associated.[15] This complication seems to occur more frequently in male patients, contrasting with the overall female gender predilection of PM/DM. Each case reviewed had concurrent ILD, suggesting that this is a risk factor for spontaneous pneumomediastinum. The overall mortality is thought to be near 34%, with almost one-fourth of cases resulting in death within 1 month of onset.[15]

### Drug-induced Pneumonitis

In patients with inflammatory myopathy, multiple different immunosuppressive agents are used, some of which can produce interstitial inflammation that is difficult to distinguish from ILD associated with the underlying disease. Methotrexate and cyclophosphamide are prime examples of medications that have been associated with drug-induced ILD.

Methotrexate-induced pneumonitis can occur at any dose and at any time during the course of treatment, although it most often occurs during the first year of therapy and usually resolves with discontinuation of the drug.[16] Cyclophosphamide-induced pneumonitis presents in 2 different ways: either as an acute pneumonitis early in the course of treatment or as a chronic, progressive process after prolonged therapy. The chronic form tends to persist or advance despite discontinuation of therapy, whereas the acute form may improve gradually after drug discontinuation.[17] Beyond methotrexate and cyclophosphamide, many of the newer antimetabolites (eg, leflunomide) and biologic agents have also been associated with pneumonitis,[18,19] effectively highlighting the complexity of pharmacologic management in IIM.

## INTERSTITIAL LUNG DISEASE

Up to 75% of patients with inflammatory myopathy develop intrinsic pulmonary involvement in the form of ILD, a complication that is largely responsible for the morbidity and mortality of this disease. ILD can present insidiously or acutely, reflecting a variety of pathologic processes/histopathologic abnormalities.

### Clinical Presentation

Most patients with ILD present with cough, dyspnea, and varying degrees of hypoxemia. This condition can develop gradually over weeks to months, or progress more rapidly with respiratory failure developing over days to weeks; in severe cases, patients present with acute respiratory distress syndrome. Overall, the relative frequency of acute versus chronically progressive disease seems to be evenly distributed in myositis-associated lung disease. ILD precedes the diagnosis of DM/PM in approximately 13% to 37.5% of patients.[4,20–22]

### Serum Biomarkers

Several clinical subsets of myositis associated with ILD exist as independent entities or as part of overlap syndromes defined by additional features of systemic lupus erythematosus, Sjögren syndrome, systemic sclerosis, or mixed connective tissue disease. In many instances, these clinical subsets are marked by antibodies directed toward various cytoplasmic and/or nuclear antigens. The nomenclature is variable, but includes myositis-associated antibodies such as ANA (52%), anti-SSA/SSB (12%), anti-U1-RNP (11%),[23] anti-PM/Scl, and anti-Ku. Although these antibodies are not specific for PM/DM and can be found in other autoimmune disorders, other antibodies are more exclusive to myositis and are therefore referred to as myositis-specific antibodies (MSAs). MSAs encompass anti–signal recognition particle complex (anti-SRP), anti–Mi-2, anti–aminoacyl transfer RNA (tRNA) synthetase (anti-ARS), anti–CADM-140/MDA-5, and anti-155/140 (transcription intermediary factor 1 [TIF1$\gamma$]) antibodies (**Table 2**).

Of the MSAs, antibodies targeting various tRNA synthetases are perhaps most strongly linked with the presence of ILD. Aminoacyl tRNA synthetases (ARSs) catalyze the binding of amino acids to corresponding transfer RNAs as part of ribosomally mediated protein translation in the cytoplasm. Although 20 different tRNA synthetases exist, only 8 have been identified as autoantibody targets to date: anti–Jo-1, anti–PL-7, anti–PL-12, anti-EJ, anti-OJ, anti-KS, anti-Zo, and anti–tyrosyl-tRNA synthetase (**Table 3**). These antibodies collectively define the antisynthetase syndrome that is marked by the variable combination of myositis, arthritis, fever, Raynaud phenomenon, mechanic's hands, and ILD.

Among patients with anti-ARS antibodies, the prevalence of ILD is estimated to be 67% to 100% depending on the particular antibody detected.[12,24,25] Although the presence of other nonsynthetase autoantibodies (such as anti-Ro52, anti–U1-RNP) is common in patients with the antisynthetase syndrome, the coexistence of multiple antisynthetase antibodies in a patient is exceedingly rare.[21,24]

Anti-Jo-1 is the most commonly identified anti-ARS antibody. It is positive in approximately 20% to 30% of patients with PM/DM, most commonly (but not exclusively) in polymyositis. This antibody specificity represents an independent predictor of ILD in this population,[26–28] because up to 90% of patients with anti–Jo-1 antibodies develop some form of ILD.[29,30] Moreover, existing studies indicate that the lung disease may be more severe in African American compared to Caucasian patients with anti–Jo-1 antibodies.[31]

| Table 2 Myositis-specific antibodies | | | |
|---|---|---|---|
| **Antibody** | **Target** | **Subset** | **Phenotype** |
| Jo-1 | Histidyl-tRNA Synthetase | PM/DM | Antisynthetase syndrome |
| CADM-140 | MDA-5 | DM | Amyopathic, ILD, cutaneous ulceration |
| SAE | SUMO | DM | ILD, dysphagia |
| Mi-2 | NuRD | DM | Shawl, V-neck, Gottron sign |
| MJ | NXP-2 | JDM | Calcinosis, ulceration |
| p155/140 | TIF1-$\gamma$ | DM, JDM | Severe skin disease, malignancy[a] |
| SRP | 72 kDa and 54 kDa subunits of SRP | PM | Severe/refractory myositis |

*Abbreviations:* JDM, juvenile dermatomyositis; MDA-5, melanocyte differentiation-associated antigen-5 (RNA helicase); NuRD, nucleosome remodeling deacetylase complex; NXP-2, nuclear matrix protein-2; SRP, signal recognition particle; SUMO, small ubiquitinlike modifier activating enzyme; TIF1-$\gamma$, transcriptional intermediary factor 1-gamma.
[a] Malignancy associated with adult DM.

**Table 3**
**Antisynthetase antibodies**

| Antisynthetase Antibodies | Target Antigen | Prevalence in IIM (%) |
|---|---|---|
| Anti–Jo-1 | Histidyl-tRNA synthetase | 20–30 |
| Anti–PL-7 | Threonyl-tRNA synthetase | <5 |
| Anti–PL-12 | Alanyl-tRNA synthetase | <5 |
| Anti-EJ | Glycyl-tRNA synthetase | <5 |
| Anti-OJ | Isoleucyl-tRNA synthetase | <5 |
| Anti-KS | Asparaginyl-tRNA synthetase | <1 |
| Anti-Zo | Phenylalanyl-tRNA synthetase | <1 |
| Anti-YRS | Tyrosyl-tRNA synthetase | <1 |

After anti–Jo-1, the next most common anti-ARS antibodies are anti–PL-7 and anti–PL-12, which are identified in another 5% of patients with the antisynthetase syndrome. Both affect women more often than men, with symptoms often manifesting in the fifth to sixth decades of life. Patients with anti–PL-7 and anti–PL-12 tend to present with a higher incidence of ILD in the absence of clinical myositis.[32] A few studies found that usual interstitial pneumonia (UIP) was more common than nonspecific interstitial pneumonia (NSIP) when histopathologic diagnosis was obtained.[33,34] Overall, because the other anti-ARS antibodies make up less than 2% of patients with the antisynthetase syndrome, little is known about their specific phenotypes; however, smaller case series highlight the association of several of these less frequently observed anti-ARS antibodies with ILD.[35–37]

Beyond these autoantibody specificities, anti–CADM-140/anti–MDA-5 antibodies are associated with a phenotype similar to the antisynthetase syndrome, with a high risk of rapidly progressive ILD.[38] Rarely found in other connective tissue disorders, anti–MDA-5 antibodies target interferon-induced helicase-1, a molecule that recognizes single-stranded RNA viruses as part of the innate immune response. Most studies show that patients with anti–MDA-5 are more likely to present with an acute-onset, rapidly progressive form of ILD, although the severity of ILD may vary in different ethnic populations.[39–42] Extrapulmonary features include absent/subclinical (amyopathic) muscle disease and striking dermatologic manifestations such as cutaneous ulcerations.[42] Overall, because of the association with severe/rapidly progressive ILD, anti–CADM-140/MDA-5 antibodies represent important serologic markers of increased mortality in patients with amyopathic dermatomyositis.[38,43]

In contrast with the aforementioned antibodies, several MSAs associated with distinct clinical syndromes portend a low risk of ILD. For example, the myositis-specific antibody anti-155/140 targets TIF1 family proteins, is present in approximately 13% to 16% of patients with DM/PM, and is highly associated with the presence of malignancy[44] – but carries a much lower risk of ILD.[28] Anti-SRP and anti–Mi-2 antibodies are also associated with a lower risk of ILD. Present in 4% of patients with myositis, anti-SRP antibodies are associated with severe muscle disease that is often poorly responsive to treatment.[45,46] In contrast, anti-Mi-2 antibodies are typically associated with diffuse, steroid-responsive skin involvement and are present in about 4% to 14% of patients with IIM, almost exclusively in dermatomyositis.[45,47]

## Nonantibody Biomarkers

As a complement to serum antibodies that define specific clinical phenotypes, researchers have also identified nonantibody biomarkers that correlate with disease activity and prognosis in certain groups. Among these, serum ferritin, KL-6, C-reactive protein (CRP), and CXCL9/10 are included. For example, hyperferritinemia is associated with a rapidly progressive form of ILD in patients with PM/DM, with levels that correlate with disease activity.[48,49] Survival rates were significantly lower when serum ferritin exceeded 1500 ng/mL in patients with acute interstitial pneumonia (AIP) and DM. Because interleukin-6, interleukin-8, and interleukin-10 play an important role in hyperferritinemia, these cytokines represent potential targets for therapeutic investigation.[48,49]

KL-6 is a mucinous high-molecular-weight glycoprotein, expressed on type 2 pneumocytes. Serum levels tend to be significantly higher in patients with PM/DM compared to healthy controls. Increased serum KL-6 levels correlated directly with the stage/severity of ILD, and inversely with measures of forced expiratory volume in 1 second (FEV1), vital capacity, total lung capacity, and DLCO (diffusion capacity (of the lung) for carbon monoxide) on pulmonary function testing.[50,51]

Richards and colleagues[30] examined serum CRP and the serum chemokines CXCL9 and CXCL10 as possible peripheral blood biomarkers of ILD in anti–Jo-1 antibody–positive patients. Comparing anti–Jo-1 antibody–positive patients with ILD to anti-SRP antibody–positive myositis controls lacking pulmonary involvement and to idiopathic pulmonary fibrosis, these investigators found that anti–Jo-1 antibody–positive patients with ILD showed significantly higher serum levels of CRP, CXCL9, and CXCL10. Moreover, among those anti–Jo-1 antibody–positive patients undergoing lung biopsy, UIP and diffuse alveolar damage (DAD) emerged as predominant histopathologic patterns. Subgroup analysis also showed that anti–Jo-1 antibody–positive patients with DAD had significantly higher levels of CXCL9 and CXCL10 compared to those with UIP, suggesting that it may be possible to distinguish histopathologic subtypes with serum biomarkers (rather than invasive procedures) before clinical decompensation.

## Histopathology

As suggested by the preceding discussion, myositis-associated ILD manifests with a spectrum of histopathologic features. In most studies, the predominant form is NSIP, accounting for 60% to 80% of cases confirmed by biopsy.[5,52] Although most remaining cases stem from cryptogenic organizing pneumonia (COP) (15%–20%) and UIP (10%–15%), a small percentage of cases involve DAD or AIP.[5,52] Among patients with the antisynthetase syndrome, individual antibody specificity does not seem to correlate with histologic pattern,[21] although several studies have indicated a higher than expected prevalence of UIP and DAD compared with nonsynthetase subgroups.[33,35] Overall, these studies must be interpreted cautiously, because the estimated prevalence of histopathologic subtypes is influenced by specific serologically/clinically defined phenotypes as well as referral bias related to disease severity.

## Imaging

Corresponding to this array of underlying histopathologic abnormalities, chest imaging represents a valuable noninvasive tool contributing to the diagnostic assessment and characterization of myositis-associated ILD. Although chest radiograph findings are less specific with abnormalities that can include basilar interstitial infiltrates in an alveolar pattern, high-resolution computed tomography (HRCT) findings are generally more informative, but highly variable, depending on the underlying histopathologic subtype of ILD. For example, the HRCT pattern associated with UIP is marked by predominant posterobasal interstitial thickening that is often patchy with reticular abnormalities, honeycombing, and traction bronchiectasis. These findings differ from NSIP, in which ground-glass opacification (GGO) is the salient feature, often associated with some evidence of fibrosis, but rarely with honeycombing or consolidation.[53] In contrast, consolidation is present in 90% of patients with COP and can be either bilateral or unilateral. Lower lungs are more frequently involved in COP, and GGO are present in about 60% of cases; the presence of reticular opacities usually indicates some degree of fibrosis and can predict a poorer response to steroids.[54] The most common computed tomography (CT) findings in AIP are bilateral, patchy regions of GGO interspersed with focal areas of relative sparing and lung nodules. Consolidation in the dependent portions of the lung is also common in AIP. In the organizing phase of DAD there can be distortion of the bronchovascular bundles and traction bronchiectasis, mainly in nondependent areas of the lung.[53]

Assessing this range of abnormalities in a retrospective study of 25 patients with myositis-associated ILD, Ikezoe and colleagues[55] found that 92% showed GGOs, 92% had linear opacities, 52% had airspace consolidation, and 16% had honeycombing. In another study, the patients were divided into acute and chronic subgroups based on their clinical presentation. The acute group had more severe respiratory symptoms, hypoxemia, and worse lung function, which collectively correlated with increased GGO and consolidation on HRCT. In contrast, the chronic subgroup manifested abnormalities characterized by predominant reticulation and honeycombing on HRCT.[20] Viewed broadly, these studies suggest that early disease may be characterized by more active inflammation in the form of consolidation and GGO that contrasts with the reticular abnormalities and honeycombing associated with more chronic/advanced forms of disease.

### Pulmonary Function Tests

Pulmonary function tests (PFTs) in myositis-associated ILD complement the data provided by imaging and histopathology, typically showing a restrictive pattern with low forced vital capacity, low total lung capacity, and diminished DLCO.[31,56] Early in the disease, patients may have normal spirometry and lung volumes with only a mildly reduced DLCO, or decreased $O_2$ saturation with 6-minute walk testing (6MWT). The latter observation highlights the value of 6MWTas a screening tool for patients with early findings on CT scan or nonspecific symptoms that may emerge more clearly in active/dynamic (rather than static) functional testing. As previously mentioned, more detailed measurement of MIF and MEF may aid in the assessment of respiratory muscle weakness, which can contribute to ventilatory failure.

### Bronchoscopy

Diagnostic bronchoscopy is not widely used in the evaluation of myositis-associated ILD. However, limited studies suggest that the bronchoalveolar fluid in myositis-associated ILD is hypercellular with a predominance of CD8+ lymphocytes.[21,57] Because these findings are not pathognomonic, many cases require an open lung biopsy to confirm the diagnosis. Nevertheless, bronchoscopy with bronchoalveolar lavage can be helpful in ruling out DAD/hemorrhage or infection in the setting of acutely worsening/new symptoms.

### Surgical Lung Biopsy

Although surgical lung biopsy may be required for more specific subclassification of myositis-associated ILD, it is not always performed, either because HRCT abnormalities are suggestive/diagnostic or because establishing the exact histopathologic diagnosis would not influence the treatment plan. Transbronchial biopsy is of limited diagnostic utility in this setting, and the risks of more invasive open lung biopsy procedures (via video-assisted thoracoscopic surgery) must always be considered when evaluating the potential value of histopathologic classification in therapeutic decision making.

### Management

Corticosteroids are the first-line therapy for ILD associated with inflammatory myopathies. One suggested regimen for moderately severe disease is prednisone 1 mg/kg by mouth daily. For severe, rapidly progressive ILD, pulse intravenous methylprednisolone 1 g daily for 3 days followed by prednisone 1 mg/kg by mouth daily[1] is often used. In general, the response to corticosteroids varies by histopathologic subtype and stage/severity of ILD; although COP generally responds to corticosteroid therapy, NSIP tends to have a variable response to steroid monotherapy, and DAD is generally refractory/relentlessly progressive even in the setting of high-dose corticosteroids.[58] Beyond histopathologic subtype, the underlying clinical/serologic phenotype seems to influence treatment responsiveness. For example, in the antisynthetase syndrome, patients respond better to corticosteroids than anti-ARS–negative patients, although they also have a higher incidence of ILD relapse. Overall, Yoshifuji and colleagues[59] found no difference in PFTs at 2 years between anti-ARS–positive and anti-ARS–negative subgroups when treated with corticosteroids alone.

As shown by this analysis as well as other studies, treatment of myositis-associated ILD often requires additional immunosuppressive medications.[59] Multiple agents have been tested, but no large randomized controlled trials exist. Mycophenolate mofetil (MMF) has proved to be safe and well tolerated for connective tissue disease–related ILD,[60] although the published experience in myositis-associated ILD remains limited. For example, in an open trial of 5 patients with myositis-associated ILD, treatment with MMF yielded no significant change in PFTs at 18-month follow-up. However, in 2 other case series involving a total of 7 patients with myositis-associated ILD, MMF treatment resulted in clinical improvement and complete resolution of HRCT findings.[22,61] In the study by Marie and colleagues[22] showing potential beneficial effects of MMF, most patients were anti–Jo-1 positive, suggesting that this serologically/clinically defined subgroup has a more favorable response. These reports collectively indicate that MMF may serve as an effective steroid-sparing agent with a favorable side effect profile (requiring less frequent monitoring compared with other agents such as cyclophosphamide), but further studies are clearly required.

Alternative second-line agents used in conjunction with prednisone include azathioprine and cyclophosphamide. In one small series of myositis-associated ILD, azathioprine showed efficacy as maintenance therapy following initial treatment with cyclophosphamide.[22] Yamasaki and colleagues[62] studied intravenous cyclophosphamide in 17 patients with myositis-associated ILD, and the mean vital capacity, HRCT lesions, and dyspnea all improved with therapy. An additional study confirmed these findings by showing that dyspnea improved in 55% of the patients treated with cyclophosphamide.[22]

The calcineurin inhibitors cyclosporine and tacrolimus are T cell–targeted therapies that have also been studied in the context of myositis-associated ILD. Takada and colleagues[63] retrospectively reviewed 53 patients with PM/DM treated with cyclo-sporin A (CsA) in addition to corticosteroids. After 4 weeks of treatment with CsA, many patients showed improvement; however, there was no clear benefit in patients with the acute, rapidly progressive form of ILD. In contrast, alternative studies have shown clinical, physiologic, and radiographic improvement through combination ther-apy with corticosteroids and CsA (with and without preceding cyclophosphamide) in the subset of patients with myositis presenting with acute/subacute interstitial pneu-monia.[64,65] However, the use of cyclosporine requires frequent monitoring of drug levels and is associated with multiorgan toxicities, often making it a less favorable treatment option.

Tacrolimus is another, potentially less toxic, calcineurin inhibitor (although still requiring frequent laboratory monitoring) that may be effective as an alternative treatment in refractory cases. Kurita and colleagues[66] retrospectively evaluated 49 patients who were treated with the combination of corticosteroids and tacroli-mus or corticosteroids alone. The tacrolimus group had significantly longer respira-tory event–free survival and disease-free survival. These findings support case series observations showing the effectiveness of tacrolimus in the treatment of ILD associated with the antisynthetase syndrome[67] and further suggest that the clinical/serologic subset represents an important determinant in the selection of therapeutic agents.

In terms of biologic agents, rituximab has been tried in some patients who had pre-viously failed multiple other therapies. For example, when given to 11 patients with the antisynthetase syndrome and refractory ILD, 7 of the 11 patients showed stabilization or improvement. Although these results provide a rationale for further study, the de-gree of immunosuppression and risk of fatal infection must be considered (1 patient died of infection in this study).[68]

### Prognosis

Patients with pulmonary complications of DM/PM follow variable clinical courses. Approximately 40% of patients experience a reduction in their functional status caused by pulmonary issues, whereas another 8% develop respiratory failure and require oxygen supplementation.[6] Some factors associated with worse prognosis include older age at onset (>55 years), symptomatic acute ILD, and abnormal PFT parameters (at diagnosis) consisting of lower forced vital capacity, vital capacity, and DLCO .[6] Beyond these parameters, HRCT findings of honeycombing/traction bronchiectasis or a histopathologic diagnosis of UIP portends a worse prognosis, as does steroid-refractory disease.[6] Although studies have shown a better overall survival in patients with myositis-associated ILD (including UIP) compared to idio-pathic pulmonary fibrosis[52] – with 85%, 75%, and 60% survival rates at 1, 3, and 5 years – ILD contributes significantly as an independent risk factor for death in pa-tients with IIM.

Given the highly negative impact of ILD on patient quality of life and survival, early identification of parenchymal lung abnormalities and determination of risk factors for disease progression are critical for selection of patients who should undergo aggres-sive medical therapy. Management of potential comorbidities such as gastroesoph-ageal reflux, pulmonary artery hypertension, and infection are equally important and suggest that patients should undergo baseline studies of esophageal function as well as serial echocardiography and pulmonary function testing. The frequency of repeat imaging has not been established, but should likely follow changes in clinical status and/or declining PFT parameters. Coupled with appropriate vaccination strategies and prophylaxis for opportunistic infections such as PCP, this rigorous management approach is likely to be required to improve patient outcomes as clinicians search for more effective therapies.

## SUMMARY/FUTURE DIRECTIONS

Over the last 10 years, understanding of the clinical characteristics, serologic markers, and treatment responsiveness of myositis-associated ILD has advanced considerably. However, based on the rarity of IIM, conducting large, randomized clinical trials comparing efficacy of different therapeutic strategies is not feasible. Therefore, future efforts should focus on the development of standardized HRCT grading schemes and other outcome measures that will permit composite evaluation of data collected through multiple centers. This collaborative approach will not only require data sharing, but also the integrated effort of multiple subspecialties, including rheumatology, pulmonology, radiology, and pathology. Aided by advances in molecular profiling (involving serologic, proteomic, and genetic markers), improved consensus regarding relevant outcome measures will deepen understanding of ILD pathophysiology and facilitate the evaluation of more rational, targeted therapies for this potentially devastating complication of IIM.

## REFERENCES

1. Hallowell R, Ascherman D, Danoff S. Pulmonary manifestations of polymyositis/dermatomyositis. Semin Respir Crit Care Med 2014;35:239–48.
2. Mills E, Mathews W. Interstitial pneumonitis in dermatomyositis. J Am Med Assoc 1956;160(17):1467–70.
3. Mimori T, Nakashima R, Hosono Y. Interstitial lung disease in myositis: clinical subsets, biomarkers, and treatment. Curr Rheumatol Rep 2012;14(3):264–74.
4. Chen IJ, Jan We YJ, Lin C, et al. Interstitial lung disease in polymyositis and dermatomyositis. Clin Rheumatol 2009;28(6):639–46.
5. Marie I, Hatron PY, Dominique S, et al. Short-term and long-term outcomes of interstitial lung disease in polymyositis and dermatomyositis: a series of 107 patients. Arthritis Rheum 2011;63(11):3439–47.
6. Marie I, Ménard J, Hachulla E, et al. Infectious complications in polymyositis and dermatomyositis: a series of 279 patients. Semin Arthritis Rheum 2011;41(1):48–60.
7. Tobin R, Pope C, Pellegrini C, et al. Increased prevalence of gastroesophageal reflux in patients with idiopathic pulmonary fibrosis. Am J Respir Crit Care Med 1998;158(6):1804–8.
8. Green H, Paul M, Vidal L, et al. Prophylaxis for pneumocystis pneumonia (PCP) in non-HIV immunocompromised patients [review]. Cochrane Database Syst Rev 2007;(18):CD005590.
9. Enomoto T, Azuma A, Matsumoto A, et al. Preventive effect of sulfamethoxasole-trimethoprim on *Pneumocystis jiroveci* pneumonia in patients with interstitial pneumonia. Intern Med 2008;47(1):15–20.
10. Mori S, Sugimoto M. *Pneumocystis jirovecii* infection: an emerging threat to patients with rheumatoid arthritis. Rheumatology (Oxford) 2012;51(12):2120–30.
11. Marie I, Hachulla E, Chérin P, et al. Opportunistic infections in polymyositis and dermatomyositis. Arthritis Rheum 2005;53(2):155–65.
12. Hervier B, Meyer A, Dieval C, et al. Pulmonary hypertension in antisynthetase syndrome: prevalence, aetiology and survival. Eur Respir J 2013;42(5):1271–82.
13. Denbow C, Lie J, Tancredi R, et al. Cardiac involvement in polymyositis: a clinicopathologic study of 20 autopsied patients. Arthritis Rheum 1979;22(10):1088–92.

14. Selva-O'Callaghan A, Sanchez-Sitjes L, Munoz-Gall X, et al. Respiratory failure due to muscle weakness in inflammatory myopathies: maintenance therapy with home mechanical ventilation. Rheumatology (Oxford) 2000;39(8):914–6.

15. Le Goff B, Chérin P, Cantagrel A, et al. Pneumomediastinum in interstitial lung disease associated with dermatomyositis and polymyositis. Arthritis Rheum 2009;61(1):108–18.

16. Imokawa S, Colby T, Leslie K, et al. Methotrexate pneumonitis: review of the literature and histopathological findings in nine patients. Eur Respir J 2000;15(2):373.

17. Malik S, Myers J, DeRemee R, et al. Lung toxicity associated with cyclophosphamide use. Two distinct patterns. Am J Respir Crit Care Med 1996;154(6):1851–6.

18. Savage RL, Highton J, Boyd IW, et al. Pneumonitis associated with leflunomide: a profile of New Zealand and Australian reports. Intern Med J 2006;36(3):162–9.

19. Hadjinicolaou AV, Nisar MK, Bhagat S, et al. Non-infectious pulmonary complications of newer biological agents for rheumatic diseases—a systematic literature review. Rheumatology (Oxford) 2011;50(12):2297–305.

20. Won Huh J, Soon Kim D, Keun Lee C, et al. Two distinct clinical types of interstitial lung disease associated with polymyositis-dermatomyositis. Respir Med 2007; 101(8):1761–9.

21. Koreeda Y, Higashimoto I, Yamamoto M, et al. Clinical and pathological findings of interstitial lung disease patients with anti-aminoacyl-tRNA synthetase autoantibodies. Intern Med 2010;49(5):361–9.

22. Marie I, Josse S, Hatron PY, et al. Interstitial lung disease in anti-Jo-1 patients with antisynthetase syndrome. Arthritis Care Res (Hoboken) 2013;65(5):800–8.

23. Love L, Leff R, Fraser D, et al. A new approach to the classification of idiopathic inflammatory myopathy: myositis-specific autoantibodies define useful homogeneous patient groups. Medicine 1991;70(6):360–74.

24. Hamaguchi Y, Fujimoto M, Matsushita T, et al. Common and distinct clinical features in adult patients with anti-aminoacyl-tRNA synthetase antibodies: heterogeneity within the syndrome. PLoS One 2013;8(4):e60442.

25. Hervier B, Benveniste O. Clinical heterogeneity and outcomes of antisynthetase syndrome. Curr Rheumatol Rep 2013;15(8):349.

26. Brouwer R, Hengstman GJ, Egberts WV, et al. Autoantibody profiles in the sera of European patients with myositis. Ann Rheum Dis 2001;60(2):116–23.

27. Mimori T, Imura Y, Nakashima R, et al. Autoantibodies in idiopathic inflammatory myopathy: an update on clinical and pathophysiological significance. Curr Opin Rheumatol 2007;19(6):523–9.

28. Solomon J, Swigris J, Brown K. Myositis-related interstitial lung disease and antisynthetase syndrome. J Bras Pneumol 2011;37(1):100–9.

29. Marie I, Hachulla E, Chérin P, et al. Interstitial lung disease in polymyositis and dermatomyositis. Arthritis Rheum 2002;47(6):614–22.

30. Richards T, Eggbeen A, Gibson K, et al. Characterization and peripheral blood biomarker assessment of anti-Jo-1 antibody-positive interstitial lung disease. Arthritis Rheum 2009;60(7):2183–92.

31. Mileti L, Strek M, Niewold T, et al. Clinical characteristics of patients with anti-Jo-1 antibodies: a single center experience. J Clin Rheumatol 2009;15(5):254–5.

32. Fischer A, Swigris JJ, du Bois, et al. Anti-synthetase syndrome in ANA and anti-Jo-1 negative patients presenting with idiopathic interstitial pneumonia. Respir Med 2009;103(11):1719–24.

33. Yousem S, Schneider F, Bi D, et al. The pulmonary histopathologic manifestations of the anti-PL7/antithreonyl transfer RNA synthetase syndrome. Hum Pathol 2014; 45(6):1199–204.

34. Kalluri M, Sahn S, Oddis C, et al. Clinical profile of anti-PL-12 autoantibody. Cohort study and review of the literature. Chest 2009;135(6):1550–6.
35. Schneider F, Yousem S, Bi D, et al. Pulmonary pathologic manifestations of anti-glycyl-tRNA synthetase (anti-EJ)-related inflammatory myopathy. J Clin Pathol 2014;67(8):678–83.
36. Kunimasa K, Arita M, Nakazawa T, et al. The clinical characteristics of two anti-OJ (anti-isoleucyl-tRNA synthetase) autoantibody-positive interstitial lung disease patients with polymyositis/dermatomyositis. Intern Med 2012;51(24): 3405–10.
37. Betteridge Z, Gunawardena H, North J, et al. Anti-synthetase syndrome: a new autoantibody to phenylalanyl transfer RNA synthetase (anti-Zo) associated with polymyositis and interstitial pneumonia. Rheumatology (Oxford) 2007;46(6): 1005–8.
38. Cao H, Pan M, Kang Y, et al. Clinical manifestations of dermatomyositis and clinically amyopathic dermatomyositis patients with positive expression of anti-melanoma differentiation-associated gene 5 antibody. Arthritis Care Res (Hoboken) 2012;64(10):1602–10.
39. Sarkar K, Weinberg C, Oddis V, et al. Seasonal influence on the onset of idiopathic inflammatory myopathies in serologically defined subgroups. Arthritis Rheum 2005;52(8):2433–8.
40. Muro Y, Suguira K, Hoshino K, et al. Epidemiologic study of clinically amyopathic dermatomyositis and anti-melanoma differentiation-associated gene 5 antibodies in central Japan. Arthritis Res Ther 2009;13(6):R214. http://dx.doi.org/10.1186/ar3547.
41. Tomohiro K, Fujikawa L, Horai Y, et al. The diagnostic utility of anti-melanoma differentiation-association gene 5 antibody testing for predicting the prognosis of Japanese patients with DM. Rheumatology (Oxford) 2012;51:1278–84.
42. Fiorentino D, Chung L, Zwerner J, et al. The mucocutaneous and systemic phenotype of dermatomyositis patients with antibodies to MDA5 (CADM-140): a retrospective study. J Am Acad Dermatol 2011;65(1):25–34.
43. Tanizawa K, Handa T, Nakashima R, et al. The prognostic value of HRCT in myositis-associated interstitial lung disease. Respir Med 2013;107(5):745–52.
44. Fujimoto M, Hamaguchi Y, Kaji K, et al. Myositis-specific anti-155/140 autoantibodies target transcription intermediary factor 1 family proteins. Arthritis Rheum 2012;64(2):513–22.
45. Hengstman G, van Engelen B, van Venrooij W. Myositis specific autoantibodies: changing insights in pathophysiology and clinical associations. Curr Opin Rheumatol 2004;16(6):692–9.
46. Kao AH, Lacomis D, Lucas M, et al. Anti-signal recognition particle autoantibody in patients with and patients without idiopathic inflammatory myopathy. Arthritis Rheum 2004;50(1):209–15.
47. Ghirardello A, Zampieri S, Iaccarino L, et al. Anti-Mi-2 antibodies. Autoimmunity 2005;38(1):79–83.
48. Kawasumi H, Gono T, Kawaguchi Y, et al. IL-6, IL-8, and IL-10 are associated with hyperferritinemia in rapidly progressive interstitial lung disease with polymyositis/dermatomyositis. Biomed Res Int 2014;2014:815245.
49. Gono T, Kawaguchi Y, Hara M, et al. Increased ferritin predicts development and severity of acute interstitial lung disease as a complication of dermatomyositis. Rheumatology (Oxford) 2010;49(7):1354–60.
50. Kubo M, Ihn H, Kikuchi K, et al. Serum KL-6 in adult patients with polymyositis and dermatomyositis. Rheumatology 2000;39(6):632–6.

51. Fathi M, Barbasso Helmers S, Lundberg I. KL-6: a serological biomarker for interstitial lung disease in patients with polymyositis and dermatomyositis. J Intern Med 2012;271(6):589–97.

52. Douglas H, Tazelaar T, Hartman R, et al. Polymyositis-dermatomyositis-associated interstitial lung disease. Am J Respir Crit Care Med 2001;164:1182–5.

53. Lynch D, Travis W, Muller N, et al. Idiopathic interstitial pneumonias: CT features. Radiology 2005;236:10–21.

54. Bouchardy L, Kuhlman J, Ball WJ, et al. CT findings in bronchiolitis obliterans organizing pneumonia (BOOP) with radiographic, clinical, and histologic correlation. J Comput Assist Tomogr 1993;17:352–7.

55. Ikezoe J, Johkoh T, Kohno N, et al. High-resolution CT findings of lung disease in patients with polymyositis and dermatomyositis. J Thorac Imaging 1996;8(4):250–9.

56. Tillie-Leblond I, Wislez M, Valeyre D, et al. Interstitial lung disease and anti-Jo-1 antibodies: difference between acute and gradual onset. Thorax 2008;63(1):53–9.

57. Sauty A, Rochat T, Schoch O, et al. Pulmonary fibrosis with predominant CD8 lymphocytic alveolitis and anti-Jo-1 antibodies. Eur Respir J 1997;10(12):2907–12.

58. Tazelaar H, Viggiano R, Pickersgill J, et al. Interstitial lung disease in polymyositis and dermatomyositis, clinical features and prognosis as correlated with histologic findings. Am Rev Respir Dis 1990;141(3):727–33.

59. Yoshifuji H, Fujii T, Kobayashi S, et al. Anti-aminoacyl-tRNA synthetase antibodies in clinical course prediction of interstitial lung disease complicated with idiopathic inflammatory myopathies. Autoimmunity 2006;39(3):233–41.

60. Swigris J, Olson A, Fischer A, et al. Mycophenolate mofetil is safe, well tolerated, and preserves lung function in patients with connective tissue disease-related interstitial lung disease. Chest 2006;130(1):30–6.

61. Morganroth PA, Kreider ME, Werth VP. Mycophenolate mofetil for interstitial lung disease in dermatomyositis. Arthritis Care Res (Hoboken) 2010;62(10):1496–501.

62. Yamasaki H, Yamada H, Yamasaki M, et al. Intravenous cyclophosphamide therapy for progressive interstitial pneumonia in patients with polymyositis/dermatomyositis. Rheumatology (Oxford) 2007;46(1):124–30.

63. Takada K, Nagasaka K, Miyasaka N. Polymyositis/dermatomyositis and interstitial lung disease: a new therapeutic approach with T-cell-specific immunosuppressants. Autoimmunity 2005;38(5):383–92.

64. Kameda H, Nagasawa H, Ogawa H, et al. Combination therapy with corticosteroids, cyclosporin A, and intravenous pulse cyclophosphamide for acute/subacute interstitial pneumonia in patients with dermatomyositis. J Clin Rheumatol 2005;32(9):1719–26.

65. Kotani T, Takeuchi T, Makino S, et al. Combination with corticosteroids and cyclosporin-A improves pulmonary function test results and HRCT findings in dermatomyositis patients with acute/subacute interstitial pneumonia. Clin Rheumatol 2011;30(8):1021–8.

66. Kurita T, Yasuda S, Oba K, et al. The efficacy of tacrolimus in patients with interstitial lung diseases complicated with polymyositis or dermatomyositis. Rheumatology (Oxford) 2015;54(1):39–44.

67. Wilkes MR, Sereika SM, Fertig N, et al. Treatment of antisynthetase-associated interstitial lung disease with tacrolimus. Arthritis Rheum 2005;52(8):2439–46.

68. Sem M, Molberg O, Lund M, et al. Rituximab treatment of the anti-synthetase syndrome: a retrospective case series. Rheumatology 2009;48(8):968–71.

69. Viguier M, Fouere S, de la Salmoniere P, et al. Peripheral blood lymphocyte subset counts in patients with dermatomyositis: clinical correlations and changes following therapy. Medicine (Baltimore) 2003;82:82–6.

# Pulmonary Manifestations of Sjögren Syndrome, Systemic Lupus Erythematosus, and Mixed Connective Tissue Disease

Isabel C. Mira-Avendano, MD[a],*, Andy Abril, MD[b]

## KEYWORDS

- Sjögren syndrome • Mixed connective tissue disease
- Systemic lupus erythematosus • Interstitial lung disease
- Connective tissue disorders

## KEY POINTS

- Systemic lupus erythematosus (SLE) has varied and frequent lung manifestations.
- Sjögren syndrome (SS) is an exocrinopathy that can affect the respiratory epithelium, leading to airway disease as the main pulmonary manifestation.
- In SLE and mixed connective tissue disease (MCTD), the main pulmonary manifestations are pleuritis and interstitial lung disease.
- The more common form of ILD in SS, SLE, and MCTD is nonspecific interstitial pneumonitis.
- Beside scleroderma, SLE and MCTD are the connective tissue diseases associated more commonly with pulmonary arterial hypertension.

## PULMONARY MANIFESTATIONS OF SJÖGREN SYNDROME
### Introduction

Sjögren syndrome (SS) is a systemic autoimmune disease characterized by lymphocytic infiltration of the exocrine glands, particularly the salivary and lacrimal glands. The term sicca syndrome is the result of dry eyes (xerophthalmia) and dry mouth (xerostomia) secondary to this involvement. It may present as a primary disease, called

Disclosures/Conflicts of Interest: No disclosures.
[a] Department of Pulmonary Medicine, Mayo Clinic, 4500 San Pablo Road, Jacksonville, FL 32224, USA; [b] Department of Rheumatology, Mayo Clinic, 4500 San Pablo Road, Jacksonville, FL 33224, USA
* Corresponding author.
E-mail address: Mira.isabel@mayo.edu

rheumatic.theclinics.com

primary SS (pSS), or be associated with other autoimmune rheumatic diseases, when is called secondary SS (sSS).[1]

The new American–European criteria have been used internationally during the last decade, but they present some limitations because they do not include the systemic manifestations, which predict prognosis. A new approach to classification has been recently proposed.[2–5]

## Physiopathology

SS is an exocrinopathy and epitheliitis characterized by lymphoproliferation and lymphocyte infiltration of glandular and nonglandular tissue. It is also a lymphocyte aggressive disease with infiltration of T and B cells into affected tissues. This lymphocyte proliferation initially contains T helper cells (CD4), B cells, and plasma cells, but in a small percentage of patients, it may continue in a dysregulated fashion to develop into lymphoma.[6,7] Extraglandular involvement has been associated with an higher incidence of autoantibodies, immune complexes, and lower complement levels, which suggests that immune complex deposition plays a role in the pathogenesis of lung disease.

## Prevalence

The population-based annual incidence of SS is 5.1 per 100,000 population, and diagnosis of pSS increases with age (18–44 years, 2.1 per 100,000 vs >75 years, 12.3 per 100,000). Survival of these patients is comparable with that of the general population.[8] There is female predominance (9:1). On the other hand, it is estimated that up to 50% of pSS patients are currently underdiagnosed, and up to 30% of patients with other autoimmune diseases can be diagnosed with sSS.[1]

Assessment of the prevalence of pulmonary involvement in SS varies considerably because of the nonstandardized diagnostic criteria and the inclusion of patients with pSS and sSS in different trials. In addition, there is no clear consensus regarding the definition of lung involvement. Most published studies indicate a prevalence of around 9 to 12%; however, if general clinical examination, pulmonary function tests (PFT), and radiologic tests are used, the prevalence increases to up to 60%.[3,8–19] Cough and dyspnea are the most common respiratory abnormalities seen in SS, and incidence of these findings increases over the duration of the illness.[20] The consensus is that patients who have secondary disease (sSS) are more likely to have more severe lung involvement because the underlying primary diseases also contribute to pulmonary pathology.[6,12] Risk factors for lung disease include hypergammaglobulinemia, lymphopenia, positive rheumatoid factor, presence of anti-Ro and anti-La antibodies, decreased forced vital capacity and forced expiratory volume in 1 second, smoking history, male gender, and advanced age at diagnosis.[3,12,19,20]

## Radiology

Chest x-rays described in early studies showed nonspecific findings.[9–12] High-resolution CT (HRCT) of the chest improved sensitivity. The main findings are signs of small airway disease, parenchymal nodules, patchy areas of ground glass attenuation, subpleural small nodules, nonseptal linear opacities, and parenchymal cysts. When the main finding is ground glass opacities, there is a predominant lower lung distribution. In contrast, pulmonary nodules are found mostly over the upper lobes.

Multiple, thin-walled air cysts are rare in other disorders and may be a crucial finding in pSS. On HRCT, they appear as well-defined, round, thin-walled airspaces that have a tendency to spread to peribronchovascular regions.[21] Overall, the HRCT features correlate well with the histopathologic findings, when biopsy is available for evaluation.[12,14–16,18,22,23]

### Pulmonary function tests

The frequency and type of physiologic impairment described in SS have varied widely, with trials showing reduced diffusion capacity for carbon monoxide (DLCO),[9,12,13,22,24] restriction,[11] and obstruction,[9,12,13,16,24] but, in general, small airway dysfunction is likely the more prevalent.[9,12,16]

In addition, almost all studies agree that the degree of physiologic damage is typically mild, as demonstrated in a 10-year follow-up study of 30 patients with pSS, in which there was evidence of improvement in DLCO in some patients, suggesting that most patients do not develop progressive disease.[22]

### Bronchoalveolar lavage and lung pathology

A few specimens of bronchoalveolar lavage have been analyzed in different series, with lymphocytosis commonly found,[12,13] and there have been some additional reports of increased numbers of neutrophils.[12,25] Transbronchial biopsies have been obtained rarely, with reported findings including amyloidosis and organizing pneumonia,[23] but it was through open lung biopsy that different patterns were defined, the most common of which were nonspecific interstitial pneumonia (NSIP), usual interstitial pneumonia (UIP), and lymphocytic interstitial pneumonia (LIP).[18,23]

### Airway disease

Airway lesions owing to glandular dysfunction and destruction may involve the trachea, bronchi, and bronchioles (distal airways), and these are the more frequent tissues affected in this disease.

**Tracheobronchial disease** Exocrine glandular lesions are more frequently associated with tracheobronchial symptoms. Sixty percent of patients in different series report having dry cough day and night. Recurrent respiratory infections (bronchitis, pneumonia) are associated with airway dysfunction in 20% of the patients with SS.[3] Proximal airway destruction may be responsible for bronchiectasis, as demonstrated by a cohort of 41 patients with pSS, who had cylindrical bronchiectasis on CT. These patients tended to be older at the time of diagnosis of SS and had a higher frequency of hiatal hernias.[26]

**Distal airway disease** Airway inflammation has been detected, and increased numbers of lymphocytes in the bronchial mucosa have been documented.[24,27] In addition, bronchiolitis secondary to extraglandular lesions may be isolated or associated with interstitial disease, such as LIP or NSIP. Follicular bronchiolitis is an uncommon bronchiolar disorder characterized by the presence of hyperplastic lymphoid follicles with reactive germinal centers distributed along bronchovascular bundles, and has been noted in SS.[28,29] The main symptoms associated with bronchiolitis are dry cough, recurrent infections, and dyspnea. Chest CT findings in bronchiolitis are characterized by signs of small airway disease with centrolobular nodules, nonseptal linear opacities, cysts, and in some cases, mild bronchiectatic changes. In addition, mosaic attenuation, which indicates obstructive bronchiolitis, may be observed and demonstrate enhancement on expiratory HRCT.[21] In cases of follicular bronchiolitis, areas of nodular centrilobular or ground glass attenuation, mild thickening of interlobular septa and bronchovascular bundles, and occasionally air cysts can be present.[21] Based on scattered data, it seems that the bronchial and bronchiolar disease in SS is benign with a stable course and good response to treatment.

### Interstitial lung disease

Interstitial lung disease (ILD) is well-described in SS.[12–16,19,20] Historically, the predominant form of ILD in pSS was deemed to be LIP,[30,31] but more recently the more common pathologic pattern identified has been NSIP, UIP, and organizing pneumonia.[23,30,32]

NSIP is characterized histologically by varying proportions of interstitial inflammation and fibrosis that are temporally uniform. The findings in CT chest images include ground glass opacities with subpleural and basilar predominance. Most patients present with dyspnea with exertion as the main symptom and restrictive pattern with decreased DLCO on PFT.[3,33,34]

UIP was documented in 17% of cases in 1 cohort.[23] It is characterized histologically by areas of fibrosis alternating with normal lung. As in NSIP, patients present with progressive dyspnea, and the PFT show restriction and decreased DLCO. The radiologic pattern shows as well predominant findings in the lower lobes, but includes reticulation and honeycombing.[33,34] Among all subtypes of ILD associated with connective tissue disease (CTD), UIP has the worst prognosis, and in fact, in this cohort of patients, when this pattern was documented in SS in this cohort of patients, they had progressive disease.[23]

SS is among the most common diseases associated with LIP.[23,32,34,35] It is characterized by diffuse interstitial infiltration of lymphocytes and plasma cells that diffusely expand the alveolar septa and small airways. The patients develop dyspnea, cough, and sometimes chest pain. PFT can present with a mixed pattern of obstruction and restriction. The chest CT reveals diffuse ground glass opacity and consolidation, with occasional thin-walled cysts, presumably owing to follicular bronchiolitis. In this last case, cystic lung disease can be documented.[21,31]

Organizing pneumonia is an entity characterized by intraluminal inflammatory debris composed of masses of fibroblasts and myofibroblasts in the alveolar ducts and airspaces with coexistent chronic inflammation of the surrounding alveoli. Clinical findings of dyspnea, associated with fever, constitutional symptoms, and lung infiltrates, could be present. Chest CT chest shows areas of consolidation.[33]

## Lymphoma

Patients with SS are at increased risk of developing non-Hodgkin lymphoma. The largest cohort of patients analyzed showed that the risk was increased either in primary pSS and sSS, but the group of patients with pSS has the greatest incidence.[36] Subsequent trials, including only patients with pSS, have shown a 16-fold increased risk for development of non-Hodgkin lymphoma compared with the general population.[37,38] Typically, these lymphomas are mostly composed of mucosa-associated lymphoid tissue (50%) and marginal zone B-cell lymphoma (40%) with low-grade malignancy. The prognosis is usually good, with an average survival rate of 65% to 90%.[3,39] Risk factors include major gland enlargement, mainly bilateral parotid, and non-exocrine manifestations, such as skin vasculitis, lymphadenopathy, and peripheral nerve involvement.[3,30,37,38] Radiologic findings in pulmonary pSS lymphoma are nonspecific; chronic alveolar opacities, reticular or reticular nodular opacities, diffuse nodular lesions, or pleural effusion have been reported. Bilateral disease is present in 25% to 50% of cases. Mediastinal involvement is not described commonly.[3] In general, LIP with unexpectedly aggressive behavior raises the question of a possible malignancy.

## Pseudolymphoma

Psuedolymphoma, also called pulmonary nodular lymphoid hyperplasia, is a benign lesion characterized by infiltration of mature polyclonal lymphocytes and plasma cells, with the presence of solitary nodule or consolidation on CT chest. It usually responds to corticosteroid therapy and progresses rarely to frank lymphoma.[30,34]

### Pulmonary amyloidosis

This is a rare complication of SS, and most of the data are based on case reports.[40] Most cases (91%) occur in pSS, with women being most frequently affected. CT of the chest shows diffuse septal, nodular infiltrates, cystic lesions, and areas of calcification.[3,30]

### Pleural involvement

Pleural involvement is rare in pSS, and its presence should prompt evaluation for the underlying etiology. Some cases of unilateral or bilateral pleuritis attributed to SS have been reported.[41] Pleural thickening has been seen as well.[13]

### Mediastinal manifestations

Mediastinal manifestations include lymphadenopathy, thymic lymphoid hyperplasia, and multilocular thymic cysts. The coexistence of these mediastinal lesions and pulmonary abnormalities may indicate pSS. On CT, these lesions are indicated by the presence of multiple nodules and increased attenuation of anterior mediastinal fat tissue.[21]

### Pulmonary hypertension

In the setting of SS, pulmonary hypertension (PH) can be the result of vasculopathy or can also be associated with lung disease, given that in the few known case series, the prevalence of lung disease has been significant.[42,43] In a trial that analyzed proven cases of PH by RHC, patients presented with advanced disease (New York Heart Association class III–IV) at the time of the diagnosis.[42] On the other hand, in a recent trial, 11 patients (all women) with pSS were found to have evidence of PH on transthoracic echocardiography and, although the diagnosis was not confirmed by RHC, these patients were significantly younger at the time of the diagnosis compared with patients without PH,[43] which suggests that perhaps more aggressive and early investigation of this complication should be considered in this population. In both studies, the patients with PH were more likely to have Raynaud phenomenon and cutaneous vasculitis, and antinuclear, anti-Ro/SSA, anti-RNP autoantibodies, positive rheumatoid factor, and hypergammaglobulinemia.[42,43]

### Treatment

The treatment for pulmonary disease in SS has not been well established, given the low number of cases evaluated. In 1996, a cohort of 11 patients was treated with azathioprine, and significant improvement in forced vital capacity after 6 months was reported compared with nontreated patients.[12] In a subsequent trial that included 18 patients, 15 received only corticosteroids and 4 received azathioprine or cyclophosphamide in addition to corticosteroids (2 were on azathioprine and 2 on cyclophosphamide), with a good response in most of cases.[23] More recently, the efficacy of rituximab in systemic manifestations of pSS was analyzed in the autoimmune and rituximab registry, and in 9 cases with pulmonary compromise (1 with bronchial involvement and 8 with ILD), its efficacy was 78%.[44] Finally, in a trial which evaluated the effect of mycophenolate mofetil on lung function in CTD–associated ILD, which included 4 patients with pSS, this medication was associated with functional improvement.[45]

## PULMONARY INVOLVEMENT IN SYSTEMIC LUPUS ERYTHEMATOSUS

Systemic lupus erythematosus (SLE) is a systemic immune disorder characterized by the production of antibodies against nuclear antigens and by immune complex deposition that can cause alteration in components of the connective tissue of multiples organs, including the lung. Although sepsis and renal disease are more common causes of death in SLE, lung disease is the predominant manifestation of the illness and an important indicator of overall prognosis, being associated with a more than 2-fold increase in mortality.[46–49]

The prevalence of lung involvement was reported as clinically significant in only 3% and pleural disease in 17% of patients at the time of diagnosis, increasing in incidence to 17% and 36%, respectively, over the course of the disease.[50]

Respiratory disease may be owing to direct involvement of the lung or pleura or as a secondary consequence of the disease affecting another organ system. Considering that the diagnosis may be difficult because of the heterogeneity of the anatomic and clinical presentations, SLE should only be considered as the specific cause of pulmonary manifestations after formally ruling out an infectious or iatrogenic disorder in these patients, who are most often immunosuppressed.[49,51]

### Pleural Disease

Pleuritis is the most common finding, with pleuritic pain occurring in 45% to 60% of the patients at some time during their course, with or without radiographically detectable effusions.[52] Pleuritis may occur along with pericarditis as a manifestation of serositis associated with active disease and is considered one of diagnostic criteria. Patients with pleuritis present with chest pain, dyspnea, cough, and fever. Pleural effusions may be either unilateral or bilateral, equally distributed between the left and right hemithorax, rarely become massive, and tend to be recurrent. Diagnostic thoracentesis is always recommended, because these patients may have effusions for many different reasons including infection, pulmonary embolism (PE), renal failure, and cardiac failure.[49,51,53,54] The pleural fluid is typically a sterile yellow or serosanguineous exudate with a variable cell count, predominantly consisting of polymorphonuclear neutrophils or lymphocytes. The glucose level can be significantly low, as in rheumatoid arthritis (but generally no less than 50 mg%), and for this reason, the glucose level cannot distinguish between effusions owing to SLE from rheumatoid arthritis, and the other criteria need to be applied. Lupus erythematosus cells can be found.[49] A high level of antinuclear antibodies (>1/160) in the fluid is strongly indicative of SLE-related pleural involvement, but only in the case of known lupus disease; a low level requires investigation of another cause. In the absence of any lupus disease, a high antibody level indicates paraneoplastic pleurisy in more than one-half of the cases.[55] Chest tube drainage, pleurodesis, and pleural biopsy are indicated rarely.[48,49,51,53,54]

The presence of small to moderate pleural effusion in the absence of symptoms does not require specific treatment. A short course of steroid therapy is generally effective in symptomatic patients, and in those with no response, antimalarial or immunosuppressive agents such as azathioprine are indicated for steroid sparing and flare prevention.[51,53,54]

### Acute Lupus Pneumonitis and Diffuse Alveolar Hemorrhage

These are uncommon, acute, life-threating complications of SLE resulting from acute injury to the alveolar–capillary unit.[56] Although any of these syndromes can be the presenting manifestation of the disease,[49,53,54] it is more common for this complication to be present during a generalized lupus flare with associated multisystem involvement, including nephritis, arthritis, and serositis, with an incidence of 1% to 4%. Diffuse alveolar hemorrhage (DAH) has a female:male ratio of approximately 6:1. The mortality associated with these complications may approach 50%.

Patients with active renal disease are at increased risk of developing DAH, which is observed in 60% to 93% of patients at the time of diagnosis.[54] An increase of DLCO of 30% or more over the baseline level or an elevation of 130% or more of the predictive value is suggestive of this diagnosis.[57] The clinical presentation in both entities is nonspecific and characterized by fever, cough, and dyspnea with hypoxemia, pleuritic chest pain, and patchy alveolar infiltrates on chest images. Hemoptysis can be present, and in the case of DAH, anemia may be present. Respiratory failure can develop, with need for mechanical ventilation.

Chest radiography and CT show unilateral or bilateral alveolar infiltrates with a ground glass or patchy consolidation appearance, usually in the lower lobes. Small pleural effusions are common. In the case of DAH, the radiologic findings can rapidly improve with bleeding cessation. Rarely, the initial chest x-ray may be normal; however, chest CT reveals the underlying lesions.[48,49,53]

Histopathologic findings are nonspecific and include alveolar wall damage and necrosis, alveolar edema or hemorrhage, hyaline membranes, and inflammatory cell infiltration.[58] Diffuse injury of the microvasculature known as capillaritis with neutrophil infiltration of alveolar septae often associated with destruction of the alveolar wall has been described in DAH.[54] An association between alkaline phosphatase and SSA/Ro antibodies has been reported, with a positive test in 80% of patients with pulmonary complications (ILD) in 2 different series.[59,60]

Bronchoalveolar lavage should be always performed, if clinically feasible. In the case of DAH, the aspirated fluid is persistently or increasingly more bloody, and the cytologic evaluation will reveal the presence of hemosiderin–laden macrophages. Lung biopsy (transbronchial or surgical) can help to establish a definite diagnosis, but it is associated with a high morbidity.[48,49,54]

Owing to the rarity of these syndromes, no prospective or controlled trials assessing therapy are available, and treatment is based in clinical experience and case reports. High-dose systemic corticosteroids such as intravenous methylprednisolone is usually given at a dose of 1 g/d as a pulse for 3 consecutive days or an equivalent prednisone dose of 1 to 2 mg/kg per day in divided doses for less critically ill patients.[16] Immunosuppressive agents such as cyclophosphamide, intravenous immunoglobulin, azathioprine, and plasmapheresis have been used in patients with poor response to steroids.[61–64] Broad spectrum antibiotics should be given and should not be suspended until infection is totally ruled out.

### Chronic Interstitial Lung Disease

ILD is less common in SLE than in other CTDs, with a clinically symptomatic process observed in 3% to 13% of patients, and although it may dominate the clinical picture in some patients, this it is rarely severe.[51,52] If imaging criteria is used, the frequency is higher, between 6% and 24% on the chest radiograph and can reach 70% on CT scans.[65]

A sequential evaluation study of pulmonary function was carried out for a duration of 2 to 7 years in 25 patients with SLE between the ages of 15 and 68 years of age, showing mild restriction and decreased DLCO at initial evaluation without significant deterioration of these values over time.[66] NSIP is likely the most common pattern in SLE patients,[67] although the real incidence of NSIP in SLE is still not well-defined.[68] LIP has been described in association with SS, and in those cases, the development of lung cysts suggest the diagnosis Organizing pneumonia pattern has been described as well in cases of SLE being related directly with the disease, or associated with infections, drug toxicity, or other systemic disorders.[69,70] For all forms of chronic ILD, corticosteroids are the first line of therapy, and then steroid-sparing agents should be considered.[45]

### Airway Disease

Airway disease is a rare, well-recognized complication of SLE. Both the upper and lower respiratory tract can be involved. Laryngeal involvement has been reported with a prevalence of 0.3% to 30% in different series[71–73] and may vary from mucosal inflammation to cricoarytenoiditis and bilateral cord paralysis. The clinical presentation depends on the severity and area of respiratory tract affected and its severity and includes hoarseness, sore throat, dry cough, dyspnea, and stridor. In contrast with rheumatoid arthritis, cricoartytenoiditis secondary to lupus is an acute process that is accompanied frequently by other lupus manifestations and has a good response to systemic steroids.[51,53,73] Lower airway involvement is characterized by obstructive pattern, reported in 6% of patients in 1 trial.[74,75] Damage of the small airways is frequent, although there is no difference when compared with the general population. However, surveillance of PFT for 2 to 7 years revealed a progressive decline in values indicating small airways damage with time, independent of smoking.[51,66,74]

## Pulmonary Arterial Hypertension

The pathogenesis of PH in CTDs in general seems to be similar to that of the primary form of the disease, with endothelial dysfunction leading to myofibroblast activation and subsequent vasoconstriction and smooth muscle hypertrophy. The prevalence of PAH in SLE ranges from 0.5% to 43%. This wide variation is seen because most studies have been conducted with small cohorts with different definitions and diagnostic methods. Data obtained through the REVEAL registry shows a 1-year survival in patients with PAH associated with SLE to be 94%, compared with scleroderma and mixed CTD (MCTD), which have the worst prognosis, with survival rates of 82% and 88%, respectively.[76,77] Treatment is similar to that for patients with primary arterial PH.[78]

## Thromboembolic Complications and Antiphospholipid Syndrome

Thrombotic events (deep venous thrombosis) with or without PE have been identified in approximately 9% of the patients with SLE and are associated commonly with disease activity. These events may or may not be associated with antiphospholid antibodies, but its presence increases the risk of thromboembolic events to 35% to 42%.[36,79]

Antiphospholipid syndrome is the association of vascular thrombosis (arterial and venous) and/or obstetric complications (early or late fetal death), the presence of lupus-type circulating anticoagulant and/or anticardiolipin antibodies and/or anti-B2GP1 antibodies, confirmed at an interval of 12 weeks.[80] Its prevalence in lupus is 30% and increases with disease progression.[79]

Catastrophic antiphospholipid syndrome is a variant that occurs in less than 1% of cases. It is characterized by rapidly progressive and diffuse microvascular occlusions in multiple organs. It carries 50% mortality. The diagnosis of catastrophic antiphospholipid syndrome is made by the presence of rapidly progressive multiorgan involvement, histopathology showing multiple vessel occlusions, and high titer antiphospholid antibodies.[81] Patients with catastrophic antiphospholipid syndrome is present in 24% of cases with pulmonary manifestations, but about 64% of patients eventually develop respiratory involvement.

Pulmonary manifestations include acute respiratory distress syndrome, PE, and DAH. The mechanism for DAH in APLS is unclear, but it is believed to be an inflammatory process precipitated by circulating antiphospholipid antibodies causing capillaritis. Treatment includes aggressive immunosuppressive therapy, including high-dose corticosteroids, intravenous immunoglobulin, and/or PE; cyclophosphamide and rituximab have been used anecdotally with some degree of success.[81–83]

## Other Clinical Manifestations

### Shrinking lung syndrome
Shrinking lung syndrome is characterized by dyspnea, respiratory muscle dysfunction, and small lung volumes on chest radiographs and PFT, with absence of pulmonary

parenchymal involvement. It is the result of possible combined diaphragmatic and chest wall dysfunction and ongoing pleural inflammation. The prevalence of shrinking lung syndrome is around 1%. Patients experience exertional dyspnea, which could be worse in the supine position. Occasionally, pleuritic chest pain can be present.[53,79] Treatment regimens including corticosteroids, with additional B2-agonist and/or theophylline. Other immunosuppressives may be indicated, but no treatment guidelines have been established.[80]

### Acute reversible hypoxemia

Acute reversible hypoxemia is a syndrome described in acutely ill, hospitalized patients with SLE and consists of hypoxemia with associated diffusion abnormalities with normal imaging studies. Hypoxemia, hypocapnia, and increased alveolo-arterial $Po_2$ gradient, are usually present. The pathogenesis is not clear but could be explained by possible leuko-occlusive vasculopathy within pulmonary capillaries induced by complement activation.[79,84,85] High-dose steroids are used with improvement detected during the initial 72 hours of treatment.

## PULMONARY MANIFESTATIONS OF MIXED CONNECTIVE TISSUE DISEASE

MCTD is an autoimmune condition with features similar to other autoimmune rheumatologic disorders. It was described for the first time in 1972 in patients who presented with mixed features of SLE, systemic sclerosis, polymyositis/dermatomyositis, and rheumatoid arthritis together with the presence of high-titer anti–U1-RNP antibodies.[86]

There have been a few classification criteria sets put together over the years, but the 2 most accepted are the Alarcon–Segovia and Khan classification criteria.[87] The Kahn criteria include serologic criteria (positive anti–U1-RNP antibodies) and the presence of swollen hands, synovitis, Raynaud phenomenon, and myositis; the Alarcon–Segovia criteria include an additional clinical manifestation, acrosclerosis. One serologic and 2 or 3 clinical criteria, depending on the author, are required for classification.[87]

Patients can present in a variety of ways, with any of the symptoms of these conditions; however, the most common manifestations are Raynaud phenomenon, hand edema (frequently described as "puffy hands"), arthralgia, and weakness owing to an inflammatory myopathy or mild sclerodactyly.

Organ involvement may be seen as well, the most common of which is pulmonary involvement, primarily PH. However, ILD, gastrointestinal manifestations such as dysphagia and dysmotility, serositis, and less commonly, cardiac and central and peripheral nervous system disease can also be seen.[88]

Because MCTD shares similar features with different CTDs, any of their pulmonary manifestations may be present; the most common manifestations are ILD, PH, and serositis; less commonly, airway disease, alveolar hemorrhage, or vasculitis can be seen.[89] It is estimated that approximately 85% of patients with MCTD may present with pulmonary involvement, most commonly ILD and PAH.[88]

### Interstitial Lung Disease

The true incidence of ILD is unknown, but a recent Scandinavian study looked at 126 patients with MCTD and found that 52% of them had abnormal HRCT changes.[90] In this study, 75% of the patients were female and all were Caucasian.

It is believed that, although pulmonary involvement is common in MCTD, in the majority of cases it is relatively mild.[91] An interesting study from Hungary followed a cohort of 201 patients with MCTD, and found through clustered analysis that patients with ILD also frequently had esophageal dysmotility and myopathy.[92] Pulmonary manifestations of MCTD are considered to be similar to systemic sclerosis, and patients should be evaluated for PAH as well.[93] The most common HRCT findings in MCTD are intralobular reticular opacities, ground glass attenuation, and nonseptal linear opacities predominating in the lower and peripheral lung fields,[89] compatible with an NSIP pattern.

### Pulmonary Arterial Hypertension

Pulmonary arterial hypertension (PAH) is a relatively common, potentially serious occurrence that carries high morbidity and mortality and is considered to be the principal cause of death in patients with MCTD.[92] The pathologic features of the pulmonary vasculature in MCTD consist of medial hypertrophy, intimal proliferation, and plexiform lesions, similar to scleroderma-associated PAH, as observed in autopsy series.[94]

Even though there are no large studies estimating the incidence of PH in MCTD, it is estimated to be around 14% to 60%, according to different series.[78,92] There seems to be a correlation between MCTD patients with PAH and the presence of anti-endothelial cell antibodies, especially if anticardiolipin antibodies and anti–U1-RNP antibodies are present concomitantly.[92]

Just as with other autoimmune rheumatologic disorders, the lesions in both IPAH and CTD-related PAH seem to be similar histologically.[77] However, the severity and prognosis of PAH in MCTD may be more favorable than other CTD, according to the REVEAL study, with better hemodynamic and right ventricular echocardiographic parameters, but a higher prevalence of pericardial effusions.[77]

Treatment of PAH in MCTD is similar to other CTDs such as scleroderma.[81]

### Pleural Effusions

Serositis in MCTD is common, with an estimated incidence varying from 6% to 50%, but pleuritic pain is only occasionally the presenting symptom; effusions are typically exudates and may be self-limiting and transient.[81]

### SUMMARY

Pulmonary manifestations in SS, SLE, and MCTD have tremendous clinical relevance, and a significant effect on prognosis, worsening the morbidity, mortality, and functional capacity of these patients. Although ILD is frequently the most recognized pulmonary manifestation in patients with CTDs, other types of involvement, such as PAH, serositis, airway disease, and pulmonary hemorrhage, can be seen and are usually quite symptomatic and often very serious. Early recognition is critical to limiting morbidity and mortality in this group of patients and emerging novel therapies may offer better treatment options in the near future.

### REFERENCES

1. Peri Y, Agmon-Levin N, Theodor E, et al. Sjogren's syndrome, the old and the new. Best Pract Res Clin Rheumatol 2012;26(1):105–17.
2. Vitali C, Bombardieri S, Jonsson R, et al. Classification criteria for Sjogren's syndrome: a revised version of the European criteria proposed by the American-European Consensus Group. Ann Rheum Dis 2002;61(6):554–8.
3. Hatron PY, Tillie-Leblond I, Launay D, et al. Pulmonary manifestations of Sjogren's syndrome. Presse Med 2011;40(1 Pt 2):e49–64.
4. Shiboski SC, Shiboski CH, Criswell L, et al. American College of Rheumatology classification criteria for Sjogren's syndrome: a data-driven, expert consensus

approach in the Sjogren's International Collaborative Clinical Alliance cohort. Arthritis Care Res (Hoboken) 2012;64(4):475–87.

5. Vitali C, Bootsma H, Bowman SJ, et al. Classification criteria for Sjogren's syndrome: we actually need to definitively resolve the long debate on the issue. Ann Rheum Dis 2013;72(4):476–8.

6. Parke AL. Pulmonary manifestations of primary Sjogren's syndrome. Rheum Dis Clin North Am 2008;34(4):907–20, viii.

7. Mavragani CP, Moutsopoulos HM. The geoepidemiology of Sjogren's syndrome. Autoimmun Rev 2010;9(5):A305–10.

8. Nannini C, Jebakumar AJ, Crowson CS, et al. Primary Sjogren's syndrome 1976–2005 and associated interstitial lung disease: a population-based study of incidence and mortality. BMJ Open 2013;3(11):e003569.

9. Constantopoulos SH, Papadimitriou CS, Moutsopoulos HM. Respiratory manifestations in primary Sjogren's syndrome. A clinical, functional, and histologic study. Chest 1985;88(2):226–9.

10. Kurumagawa T, Kobayashi H, Motoyoshi K. Potential involvement of subclinical Sjogren's syndrome in various lung diseases. Respirology 2005;10(1):86–91.

11. Papathanasiou MP, Constantopoulos SH, Tsampoulas C, et al. Reappraisal of respiratory abnormalities in primary and secondary Sjogren's syndrome. A controlled study. Chest 1986;90(3):370–4.

12. Deheinzelin D, Capelozzi VL, Kairalla RA, et al. Interstitial lung disease in primary Sjogren's syndrome. Clinical-pathological evaluation and response to treatment. Am J Respir Crit Care Med 1996;154(3 Pt 1):794–9.

13. Gardiner P, Ward C, Allison A, et al. Pleuropulmonary abnormalities in primary Sjogren's syndrome. J Rheumatol 1993;20(5):831–7.

14. Franquet T, Gimenez A, Monill JM, et al. Primary Sjogren's syndrome and associated lung disease: CT findings in 50 patients. AJR Am J Roentgenol 1997;169(3): 655–8.

15. Koyama M, Johkoh T, Honda O, et al. Pulmonary involvement in primary Sjogren's syndrome: spectrum of pulmonary abnormalities and computed tomography findings in 60 patients. J Thorac Imaging 2001;16(4):290–6.

16. Uffmann M, Kiener HP, Bankier AA, et al. Lung manifestation in asymptomatic patients with primary Sjogren syndrome: assessment with high resolution CT and pulmonary function tests. J Thorac Imaging 2001;16(4):282–9.

17. Garcia-Carrasco M, Ramos-Casals M, Rosas J, et al. Primary Sjogren syndrome: clinical and immunologic disease patterns in a cohort of 400 patients. Medicine (Baltimore) 2002;81(4):270–80.

18. Shi JH, Liu HR, Xu WB, et al. Pulmonary manifestations of Sjogren's syndrome. Respiration 2009;78(4):377–86.

19. Yazisiz V, Arslan G, Ozbudak IH, et al. Lung involvement in patients with primary Sjogren's syndrome: what are the predictors? Rheumatol Int 2010;30(10):1317–24.

20. Palm O, Garen T, Berge Enger T, et al. Clinical pulmonary involvement in primary Sjogren's syndrome: prevalence, quality of life and mortality–a retrospective study based on registry data. Rheumatology (Oxford) 2013;52(1):173–9.

21. Egashira R, Kondo T, Hirai T, et al. CT findings of thoracic manifestations of primary Sjogren syndrome: radiologic-pathologic correlation. Radiographics 2013; 33(7):1933–49.

22. Davidson BK, Kelly CA, Griffiths ID. Ten year follow up of pulmonary function in patients with primary Sjogren's syndrome. Ann Rheum Dis 2000;59(9):709–12.

23. Parambil JG, Myers JL, Lindell RM, et al. Interstitial lung disease in primary Sjogren syndrome. Chest 2006;130(5):1489–95.

24. Papiris SA, Maniati M, Constantopoulos SH, et al. Lung involvement in primary Sjogren's syndrome is mainly related to the small airway disease. Ann Rheum Dis 1999;58(1):61–4.

25. Meyer KC, Raghu G, Baughman RP, et al. An official American Thoracic Society clinical practice guideline: the clinical utility of bronchoalveolar lavage cellular analysis in interstitial lung disease. Am J Respir Crit Care Med 2012;185(9): 1004–14.

26. Soto-Cardenas MJ, Perez-De-Lis M, Bove A, et al. Bronchiectasis in primary Sjogren's syndrome: prevalence and clinical significance. Clin Exp Rheumatol 2010;28(5):647–53.

27. Papiris SA, Saetta M, Turato G, et al. CD4-positive T-lymphocytes infiltrate the bronchial mucosa of patients with Sjogren's syndrome. Am J Respir Crit Care Med 1997;156(2 Pt 1):637–41.

28. Ryu JH, Myers JL, Swensen SJ. Bronchiolar disorders. Am J Respir Crit Care Med 2003;168(11):1277–92.

29. Aerni MR, Vassallo R, Myers JL, et al. Follicular bronchiolitis in surgical lung biopsies: clinical implications in 12 patients. Respir Med 2008;102(2):307–12.

30. Kreider M, Highland K. Pulmonary involvement in Sjogren syndrome. Semin Respir Crit Care Med 2014;35(2):255–64.

31. Stojan G, Baer AN, Danoff SK. Pulmonary manifestations of Sjogren's syndrome. Curr Allergy Asthma Rep 2013;13(4):354–60.

32. Ito I, Nagai S, Kitaichi M, et al. Pulmonary manifestations of primary Sjogren's syndrome: a clinical, radiologic, and pathologic study. Am J Respir Crit Care Med 2005;171(6):632–8.

33. Sarkar PK, Patel N, Furie RA, et al. Pulmonary manifestations of primary Sjogren's syndrome. Indian J Chest Dis Allied Sci 2009;51(2):93–101.

34. Cha SI, Fessler MB, Cool CD, et al. Lymphoid interstitial pneumonia: clinical features, associations and prognosis. Eur Respir J 2006;28(2):364–9.

35. Liebow AA, Carrington CB. Diffuse pulmonary lymphoreticular infiltrations associated with dysproteinemia. Med Clin North Am 1973;57(3):809–43.

36. Kauppi M, Pukkala E, Isomaki H. Elevated incidence of hematologic malignancies in patients with Sjogren's syndrome compared with patients with rheumatoid arthritis (Finland). Cancer Causes Control 1997;8(2):201–4.

37. Voulgarelis M, Dafni UG, Isenberg DA, et al. Malignant lymphoma in primary Sjogren's syndrome: a multicenter, retrospective, clinical study by the European Concerted Action on Sjogren's Syndrome. Arthritis Rheum 1999;42(8):1765–72.

38. Theander E, Henriksson G, Ljungberg O, et al. Lymphoma and other malignancies in primary Sjogren's syndrome: a cohort study on cancer incidence and lymphoma predictors. Ann Rheum Dis 2006;65(6):796–803.

39. Hansen LA, Prakash UB, Colby TV. Pulmonary lymphoma in Sjogren's syndrome. Mayo Clin Proc 1989;64(8):920–31.

40. Rajagopala S, Singh N, Gupta K, et al. Pulmonary amyloidosis in Sjogren's syndrome: a case report and systematic review of the literature. Respirology 2010; 15(5):860–6.

41. Teshigawara K, Kakizaki S, Horiya M, et al. Primary Sjogren's syndrome complicated by bilateral pleural effusion. Respirology 2008;13(1):155–8.

42. Launay D, Hachulla E, Hatron PY, et al. Pulmonary arterial hypertension: a rare complication of primary Sjogren syndrome: report of 9 new cases and review of the literature. Medicine (Baltimore) 2007;86(5):299–315.

43. Kobak S, Kalkan S, Kirilmaz B, et al. Pulmonary arterial hypertension in patients with primary Sjogren's syndrome. Autoimmune Dis 2014;2014:710401.

44. Gottenberg JE, Cinquetti G, Larroche C, et al. Efficacy of rituximab in systemic manifestations of primary Sjogren's syndrome: results in 78 patients of the auto-immune and rituximab registry. Ann Rheum Dis 2013;72(6):1026–31.

45. Fischer A, Brown KK, Du Bois RM, et al. Mycophenolate mofetil improves lung function in connective tissue disease-associated interstitial lung disease. J Rheumatol 2013;40(5):640–6.

46. Travis WD, Colby TV, Koss MN, et al. Non-neoplastic disorders of the lower respiratory tract. 1st edition. AFIP Atlas of Nontumor Pathology. Washington (DC): American Registry of Pathology and the Armed Forces Institute of Pathology; 2002.

47. Kim JS, Lee KS, Koh EM, et al. Thoracic involvement of systemic lupus erythematosus: clinical, pathologic, and radiologic findings. J Comput Assist Tomogr 2000; 24(1):9–18.

48. Murin S, Wiedemann HP, Matthay RA. Pulmonary manifestations of systemic lupus erythematosus. Clin Chest Med 1998;19(4):641–65, viii.

49. Orens JB, Martinez FJ, Lynch JP 3rd. Pleuropulmonary manifestations of systemic lupus erythematosus. Rheum Dis Clin North Am 1994;20(1):159–93.

50. Cervera R, Khamashta MA, Font J, et al. Systemic lupus erythematosus: clinical and immunologic patterns of disease expression in a cohort of 1,000 patients. The European Working Party on systemic lupus erythematosus. Medicine (Baltimore) 1993;72(2):113–24.

51. Carmier D, Marchand-Adam S, Diot P, et al. Respiratory involvement in systemic lupus erythematosus. Rev Mal Respir 2008;25(10):1289–303.

52. Keane MP, Lynch JP 3rd. Pleuropulmonary manifestations of systemic lupus erythematosus. Thorax 2000;55(2):159–66.

53. Memet B, Ginzler EM. Pulmonary manifestations of systemic lupus erythematosus. Semin Respir Crit Care Med 2007;28(4):441–50.

54. Torre O, Harari S. Pleural and pulmonary involvement in systemic lupus erythematosus. Presse Med 2011;40(1 Pt 2):e19–29.

55. Wang DY, Yang PC, Yu WL, et al. Serial antinuclear antibodies titre in pleural and pericardial fluid. Eur Respir J 2000;15(6):1106–10.

56. Wiedemann HP, Matthay RA. Pulmonary manifestations of systemic lupus erythematosus. J Thorac Imaging 1992;7(2):1–18.

57. Ewan PW, Jones HA, Rhodes CG, et al. Detection of intrapulmonary hemorrhage with carbon monoxide uptake. Application in Goodpasture's syndrome. N Engl J Med 1976;295(25):1391–6.

58. Inoue T, Kanayama Y, Ohe A, et al. Immunopathologic studies of pneumonitis in systemic lupus erythematosus. Ann Intern Med 1979;91(1):30–4.

59. Boulware DW, Hedgpeth MT. Lupus pneumonitis and anti-SSA(Ro) antibodies. J Rheumatol 1989;16(4):479–81.

60. Mochizuki T, Aotsuka S, Satoh T. Clinical and laboratory features of lupus patients with complicating pulmonary disease. Respir Med 1999;93(2):95–101.

61. Matthay RA, Schwarz MI, Petty TL, et al. Pulmonary manifestations of systemic lupus erythematosus: review of twelve cases of acute lupus pneumonitis. Medicine (Baltimore) 1975;54(5):397–409.

62. Isbister JP, Ralston M, Hayes JM, et al. Fulminant lupus pneumonitis with acute renal failure and RBC aplasia. Successful management with plasmapheresis and immunosuppression. Arch Intern Med 1981;141(8):1081–3.

63. Winder A, Molad Y, Ostfeld I, et al. Treatment of systemic lupus erythematosus by prolonged administration of high dose intravenous immunoglobulin: report of 2 cases. J Rheumatol 1993;20(3):495–8.

64. Eiser AR, Shanies HM. Treatment of lupus interstitial lung disease with intravenous cyclophosphamide. Arthritis Rheum 1994;37(3):428–31.
65. Fenlon HM, Doran M, Sant SM, et al. High-resolution chest CT in systemic lupus erythematosus. AJR Am J Roentgenol 1996;166(2):301–7.
66. Eichacker PQ, Pinsker K, Epstein A, et al. Serial pulmonary function testing in patients with systemic lupus erythematosus. Chest 1988;94(1):129–32.
67. Devaraj A, Wells AU, Hansell DM. Computed tomographic imaging in connective tissue diseases. Semin Respir Crit Care Med 2007;28(4):389–97.
68. Tansey D, Wells AU, Colby TV, et al. Variations in histological patterns of interstitial pneumonia between connective tissue disorders and their relationship to prognosis. Histopathology 2004;44(6):585–96.
69. Gammon RB, Bridges TA, al-Nezir H, et al. Bronchiolitis obliterans organizing pneumonia associated with systemic lupus erythematosus. Chest 1992;102(4):1171–4.
70. Takada H, Saito Y, Nomura A, et al. Bronchiolitis obliterans organizing pneumonia as an initial manifestation in systemic lupus erythematosus. Pediatr Pulmonol 2005;40(3):257–60.
71. Langford CA, Van Waes C. Upper airway obstruction in the rheumatic diseases. Rheum Dis Clin North Am 1997;23(2):345–63.
72. Smith GA, Ward PH, Berci G. Laryngeal lupus erythematosus. J Laryngol Otol 1978;92(1):67–73.
73. Teitel AD, MacKenzie CR, Stern R, et al. Laryngeal involvement in systemic lupus erythematosus. Semin Arthritis Rheum 1992;22(3):203–14.
74. Andonopoulos AP, Constantopoulos SH, Galanopoulou V, et al. Pulmonary function of nonsmoking patients with systemic lupus erythematosus. Chest 1988;94(2):312–5.
75. Prabu A, Patel K, Yee CS, et al. Prevalence and risk factors for pulmonary arterial hypertension in patients with lupus. Rheumatology (Oxford) 2009;48(12):1506–11.
76. Badesch DB, Raskob GE, Elliott CG, et al. Pulmonary arterial hypertension: baseline characteristics from the REVEAL Registry. Chest 2010;137(2):376–87.
77. Chung L, Liu J, Parsons L, et al. Characterization of connective tissue disease-associated pulmonary arterial hypertension from REVEAL: identifying systemic sclerosis as a unique phenotype. Chest 2010;138(6):1383–94.
78. Ahmed S, Palevsky HI. Pulmonary arterial hypertension related to connective tissue disease: a review. Rheum Dis Clin North Am 2014;40(1):103–24.
79. Pego-Reigosa JM, Medeiros DA, Isenberg DA. Respiratory manifestations of systemic lupus erythematosus: old and new concepts. Best Pract Res Clin Rheumatol 2009;23(4):469–80.
80. Henderson LA, Loring SH, Gill RR, et al. Shrinking lung syndrome as a manifestation of pleuritis: a new model based on pulmonary physiological studies. J Rheumatol 2013;40(3):273–81.
81. Bull TM, Fagan KA, Badesch DB. Pulmonary vascular manifestations of mixed connective tissue disease. Rheum Dis Clin North Am 2005;31(3):451–64, vi.
82. Sciascia S, Lopez-Pedrera C, Roccatello D, et al. Catastrophic Antiphospholipid syndrome (CAPS). Best Pract Res Clin Rheumatol 2012;26:535–41.
83. Cartin-Ceba R, Peikert T, Ashrani AI, et al. Primary antiphospholipid syndrome–associated diffuse alveolar hemorrhage. Arthritis Care Res (Hoboken) 2014;66(2):301–10.
84. Miyakis S, Lockshin MD, Atsumi T, et al. International consensus statement on an update of the classification criteria for definite antiphospholipid syndrome (APS). J Thromb Haemost 2006;4(2):295–306.

85. Abramson SB, Dobro J, Eberle MA, et al. Acute reversible hypoxemia in systemic lupus erythematosus. Ann Intern Med 1991;114(11):941–7.
86. Sharp GC, Irvin WS, Tan EM, et al. Mixed connective tissue disease–an apparently distinct rheumatic disease syndrome associated with a specific antibody to an extractable nuclear antigen (ENA). Am J Med 1972;52(2):148–59.
87. Alarcon-Segovia D, Cardiel MH. Comparison between 3 diagnostic criteria for mixed connective tissue disease. Study of 593 patients. J Rheumatol 1989; 16(3):328–34.
88. Ortega-Hernandez OD, Shoenfeld Y. Mixed connective tissue disease: an overview of clinical manifestations, diagnosis and treatment. Best Pract Res Clin Rheumatol 2012;26(1):61–72.
89. Hant FN, Herpel LB, Silver RM. Pulmonary manifestations of scleroderma and mixed connective tissue disease. Clin Chest Med 2010;31(3):433–49.
90. Gunnarsson R, Aalokken TM, Molberg O, et al. Prevalence and severity of interstitial lung disease in mixed connective tissue disease: a nationwide, cross-sectional study. Ann Rheum Dis 2012;71(12):1966–72.
91. Gutsche M, Rosen GD, Swigris JJ. Connective tissue disease-associated interstitial lung disease: a review. Curr Respir Care Rep 2012;1:224–32.
92. Szodoray P, Hajas A, Kardos L, et al. Distinct phenotypes in mixed connective tissue disease: subgroups and survival. Lupus 2012;21(13):1412–22.
93. Olson AL, Brown KK, Fischer A. Connective tissue disease-associated lung disease. Immunol Allergy Clin North Am 2012;32(4):513–36.
94. Hosoda Y, Suzuki Y, Takano M, et al. Mixed connective tissue disease with pulmonary hypertension: a clinical and pathological study. J Rheumatol 1987;14(4): 826–30.

# Management of Connective Tissue Disease–associated Interstitial Lung Disease

Sandra Chartrand, MD, FRCPC[a,b], Aryeh Fischer, MD[c],*

## KEYWORDS

- Connective tissue disease • Collagen vascular disease • Interstitial lung disease
- Interstitial pneumonia • Pulmonary fibrosis • Treatment • Management

## KEY POINTS

- Connective tissue disease (CTD)–associated interstitial lung disease (ILD) reflects a heterogeneous spectrum of diverse CTDs and a variety of patterns of interstitial pneumonia. Other than a few controlled trials in scleroderma-ILD, there are few studies to reliably inform an evidence-based approach to managing CTD-ILD, and, in general, clinicians are left with experience-based approaches.
- The management of CTD-ILD is limited to cases with progressive and/or clinically significant disease.
- Immunosuppression with corticosteroids and cytotoxic medications are the mainstay of pharmacologic treatment.
- Extrathoracic manifestations of the CTD need to be assessed and may also affect choice and intensity of immunosuppressive therapies.
- Nonpharmacologic approaches to treatment should be considered for each patient with CTD-ILD.

Disclosure: A. Fischer serves as a paid consultant for Actelion Pharmaceuticals, Gilead Sciences, InterMune, Boehringer-Ingelheim and Seattle Genetics; S. Chartrand received bursary funding from Fondation de l'Hôpital Maisonneuve-Rosemont and Bourse de perfectionnement du Programme de rhumatologie de l'Université de Montréal - Abbvie.

[a] Department of Medicine, National Jewish Health, University of Colorado School of Medicine, 1400 Jackson Street, Denver, CO 80206, USA; [b] Department of Medicine, Rheumatology Clinic, Hôpital Maisonneuve-Rosemont, Université de Montréal, 5415 Boulevard de l'Assomption, Montréal, Québec H1T 2M4, Canada; [c] Department of Medicine, National Jewish Health, University of Colorado School of Medicine, 1400 Jackson Street, G07, Denver, CO 80206, USA
* Corresponding author.
E-mail address: fischera@njhealth.org

## INTRODUCTION

Although connective tissue disease (CTD)–associated interstitial lung diseases (ILDs) are sometimes considered a homogeneous entity (such as in this and many other articles), the spectrum of CTD-ILD reflects a heterogeneous category of diseases comprising the different CTDs along with the various interstitial pneumonia (IP) patterns. It remains to be determined whether the approach to management of one type of CTD-ILD (eg, systemic sclerosis [SSc]–nonspecific IP [NSIP]) can be applied to other forms of CTD-ILD (eg, rheumatoid arthritis [RA]–usual IP [UIP] or idiopathic inflammatory myositis [IIM]–organizing pneumonia [OP]). This article discusses our approach to the pharmacologic and nonpharmacologic therapeutic strategies for the spectrum of CTD-ILD.

## GENERAL PRINCIPLES

A fundamental principle pertinent to CTD-ILD is that many patients do not require immunosuppressive therapy targeting the ILD. In many cases, immunosuppressive treatment is needed for the extrathoracic inflammatory disease features (eg, synovitis or myositis) but not the ILD. Given the high prevalence of subclinical ILD in CTDs, it is crucial to determine the degree of respiratory impairment in all patients with CTD-ILD (see article by Ryerson elsewhere in this issue). The decision to treat CTD-ILD is often based on whether the patient is clinically impaired by the ILD; whether the ILD is progressive by symptoms, physiology, and/or imaging; and what extrathoracic features require therapy.

## MANAGEMENT OF EXTRATHORACIC MANIFESTATIONS

Traditional and biologic disease modifying antirheumatic drugs (DMARDs) are commonly used to treat the extrathoracic manifestations of the CTD, particularly synovitis and myositis. However, there is also evidence that some of these therapies,[1] methotrexate (MTX) in particular,[2] have the potential for causing pneumonitis. Those with prior lung involvement are possibly more susceptible.[3] In general, because of its potential for lung toxicity, and because it is often difficult to distinguish MTX-pneumonitis from a flare of underlying ILD, we tend to avoid or remove MTX in our patients with CTD-ILD. The biologic DMARDs have become a mainstay in rheumatology practice, and have shown a high degree of efficacy for synovitis, myositis, ocular aspects, and cutaneous aspects of RA and other CTDs.[4,5] There has been some evidence based on case reports, retrospective studies, and postmarketing surveillance that biologic DMARDs, particularly the anti–tumor necrosis factor (TNF) class, may be associated with an increased risk of pneumonitis.[1,6–8] However, because no prospective controlled data exist and there is an appreciation that multiple variables, including the underlying CTD, are associated with ILD development, progression, or exacerbation, we suggest that these agents be used with caution in patients with CTD-ILD[1,9–11] and other treatment options prioritized when possible. We frequently use the spectrum of biologic DMARDs in our patients with CTD-ILD to manage the extrathoracic manifestations and find that these agents often have minimal, if any, impact on the ILD. When both ILD and extrathoracic manifestations require treatment, we combine an agent to target the ILD (eg, azathioprine [AZA] or mycophenolate mofetil [MMF]) with a biologic DMARD (eg, etanercept or rituximab [RTX]) to target the synovitis or myositis.

## PHARMACOLOGIC THERAPY

For those individuals with CTD-ILD in whom the ILD has been deemed to be clinically significant and progressive, pharmacologic treatment with immunosuppression is judged an appropriate step in management (**Fig. 1**). There are few data to adequately inform the discussion on management strategies for CTD-ILD, the only controlled data being limited to 2 clinical trials in SSc-ILD. As such, much of the management of the spectrum of CTD-ILD is left to experience-based rather than evidence-based practice.

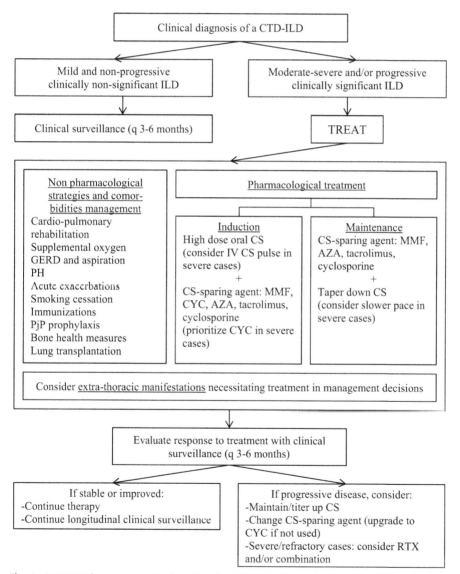

**Fig. 1.** Suggested management algorithm for CTD-ILD. CS, corticosteroids; CYC, cyclophosphamide; GERD, gastroesophageal reflux disease; IV, intravenous; PH, pulmonary hypertension; PjP, *Pneumocystis jiroveci* pneumonia.

When considering the general approach to the management of CTD-ILD, we consider the concept of induction followed by maintenance therapy, similar to the approach to systemic vasculitis. Induction therapy may require higher dosing of corticosteroids (CSs) along with short-term use of a more potent (and potentially more toxic) agent such as cyclophosphamide (CYC) followed by a maintenance regimen with a less toxic agent (such as AZA or MMF) and CS tapering. In addition, because of the often-poor prognosis associated with ILD, the ability to stabilize disease is considered a successful outcome, and, as such, setting expectations with patients and having informed discussions about goals of therapy can be helpful.

### Corticosteroids

CS therapy is the cornerstone of induction therapy in most forms of CTD-ILD in which immunosuppressive therapy is deemed to be necessary.[12,13] Considering that long-term immunosuppression is typically indicated, CS therapy is usually combined with a CS-sparing agent. We tend to initiate CSs at a dose of 0.5 to 1.0 mg/kg/d of prednisone equivalent. Depending on the clinical response and tolerability of the CS and the secondary agent, we often slowly taper the CS to attain a daily dose of 10 mg of prednisone equivalent between the fourth and sixth months of therapy, and hope for tapering off altogether when clinically feasible. No tapering regimen has been studied or proved to be more effective. A notable exception to CS use is in SSc-ILD, in which moderate to high doses of CSs are traditionally considered a risk for SSc renal crisis.[14] In SSc-ILD, we aim to keep the prednisone dose less than or equal to 15 mg/d. In our experience, there are clinical scenarios for which more intense use of CSs should be considered: acute IP, cellular NSIP or OP that may be more reversible with more intense up-front dosing of CS followed by a prolonged taper, or the NSIP encountered in patients with antisynthetase syndrome. In these cases, a pulse-dose course of intravenous (IV) methylprednisolone (500–1000 mg IV for 3 days followed by weekly pulses of 250–1000 mg IV for several weeks) concomitantly with daily oral CS at 1 mg/kg of prednisone equivalent should be considered.

The role of CSs (or any immunosuppressive agent) in patients with the UIP pattern of lung injury may be controversial. For those with idiopathic UIP (ie, the clinical scenario of idiopathic pulmonary fibrosis [IPF]), immunosuppression with the combination of CS and CYC has been proved to be ineffective.[15] Furthermore, recent data suggest that the combination of AZA, CS, and N-acetylcysteine for the treatment of IPF may lead to an increase risk of hospitalization and mortality.[16] However, such data are limited to IPF and, in our opinion, should not be extended to UIP associated with CTD. We tend to treat our patients with CTD-UIP with immunosuppression and this usually includes an initial course of CS. Further studies are needed to better guide the role of CSs in CTD-ILD in general and with UIP in particular.

### Cyclophosphamide

CYC, one of the most potent CS-sparing immunosuppressive medications, is often used to treat a variety of organ-threatening CTD manifestations. Small prospective[17–19] and retrospective[20,21] studies have suggested that the use of CYC in CTD-ILD, and SSc-ILD in particular, may lead to stabilization or improvement in lung function. In practice, CYC is often considered the first line of therapy for the most severe forms of CTD-ILD. CYC is the only agent for which there are controlled clinical trial data in CTD-ILD, but those data are limited to SSc-ILD and these studies only show modest effects of CYC.

In the Scleroderma Lung Study (SLS),[22] 158 subjects were randomized to oral CYC less than or equal to 2 mg/kg/d or placebo for 12 months. The primary end point was change in forced vital capacity (FVC). The cohort comprised subjects with SSc with evidence of active ILD by bronchoalveolar lavage or thoracic high-resolution computed tomography (HRCT) scan, early disease (first non-Raynaud symptom within 7 years), an FVC of 45% to 85% of predicted, and at least moderate exertional dyspnea. Subjects with a lung diffusion capacity for carbon monoxide (DLco) less than 30% of predicted, tobacco use in the prior 6 months, or any other significant pulmonary disease were excluded. The subjects were mostly women (70.3%) with a mean age of $47.9 \pm 1.0$ years and 59.5% had diffuse cutaneous SSc (dcSSc). The baseline mean FVC was $68.1\% \pm 1.0\%$ of predicted and DLco was $47.2\% \pm 1.1\%$ of predicted. The FVC difference ($\Delta$FVC) at 12 months was +2.53% of predicted ($P<.03$) in favor of the CYC group, remaining significant at 18 months from time of CYC initiation. However, by 24 months from CYC initiation, the treated group had regressed to FVC measures similar to the placebo arm.[23] Subjects with more restrictive disease (FVC, <70% of predicted),[23] higher fibrosis scores on thoracic HRCT scan, or more skin thickening had a more robust response to CYC (FVC at 18 months from baseline, +5.10% with CYC vs −4.71% with placebo; $\Delta$FVC, +9.81%; $P<.001$).[24]

The Fibrosing Alveolitis in Scleroderma Trial (FAST)[25] randomized 22 subjects to IV CYC 600 mg/m$^2$ monthly for the first 6 months followed by AZA 2.5 mg/kg/d with background oral prednisolone 20 mg on alternate days compared with placebo (n = 23). Subjects were mostly women with limited cutaneous SSc. The $\Delta$FVC in the active treatment group (FVC$_0$, $80.1\% \pm 10.3\%$ of predicted and FVC$_{12}$, $82.5\% \pm 11.3\%$ of predicted) compared with the placebo group (FVC$_0$, $81.0\% \pm 18.8\%$ of predicted and FVC$_{12}$, $78.0\% \pm 21.6\%$ of predicted) showed a trend toward statistical significance ($\Delta$FVC, +4.19% between groups; $P = .08$). The $\Delta$FVC was more favorable in FAST than in SLS (+4.2% vs +2.5%, respectively) but the smaller number of subjects in FAST (n = 45) compared with SLS (n − 158) affected the ability to achieve statistical significance.

In our opinion, the results from SLS and FAST have diminished enthusiasm for the use of CYC. Although modest improvements were noted in FVC, with its substantial toxicity (bone marrow suppression, infection risk, malignancy risk), its short-term and long-term use is tempered in SSc-ILD and in all forms of CTD-ILD.

The role of CYC in other forms of CTD-ILD is based on retrospective studies. In a study of 46 patients with IIM-ILD resistant to CSs, 24 were subsequently treated with oral CYC.[26] At 6 months, the $\Delta$FVC was +8.0%, the DLco difference ($\Delta$DLco) was +5.0%, and the prednisone dose was reduced from 40 mg/d to 10 mg/d. In another report by Yamasaki and colleagues,[27] 8 of 17 patients had greater than 10% improvement of vital capacity (VC) and 9 of 17 had greater than 10-point reduction in their thoracic HRCT scan scores after 6 months of treatment with CYC.

We tend to use CYC for the spectrum of CTD-ILD when the disease is severe or rapidly progressive. Because of the better safety profile of the monthly IV form compared with daily oral administration, we tend to infuse CYC monthly, generally for at least 6 months but rarely for more than 12 months. After the course of CYC, we tend to switch to a less toxic agent (eg, AZA or MMF) for longer-term maintenance therapy.

### Azathioprine

AZA is a commonly used medication for the treatment of CTD-ILD. However, other than as used in FAST, the data for AZA are limited to small and retrospective series.

Studies using AZA as a maintenance therapy following 6 months of IV CYC in SSc-ILD report contradictory data.[25,28] Less well studied as an induction agent, AZA in SSc-ILD has been retrospectively assessed in 14 patients,[29] 8 treated for 12 months and 7 for 18 months. With a baseline FVC of 54.3% ± 3.5% of predicted, 5 patients had an increase of greater than 10% and 3 stayed within 10% of their baseline at 12 months. Another recent series in SSc-ILD compared 15 patients receiving AZA (1.5–2 mg/kg/d) as an induction agent with 21 patients with oral CYC (up to 2 mg/kg/d) for 6 months with low-dose prednisolone (≤10 mg).[30] The FVCs at baseline and 12 months after treatment in AZA-treated patients were 62.8% ± 9.8% of predicted and 71.1% ± 20.9% of predicted, respectively (ΔFVC, +7.6% ± 13.1%; $P$ = .05), and in CYC-treated patients were 59.5% ± 10.7% of predicted and 63.1% ± 16.2% of predicted (ΔFVC, +2.9% ± 11.5%; $P$ = .19). In the retrospective study by Mira-Avendano and colleagues[26] of 46 patients with IIM-ILD resistant to CSs, 13 were treated with AZA. At 6 months, the ΔFVC was −4.0%, the ΔDLco was +1.0%, and the prednisone dose was reduced from 40 mg/d to 13 mg/d. In a cohort of Sjögren syndrome–ILD with multiple IP patterns, 11 patients were treated with AZA for 6 months: 7 had an increase of their FVC by greater than 10% compared with none in the 9 nontreated patients ($P$<.05).[31]

In general, we find AZA to be a well-tolerated therapy and plausibly effective CS-sparing agent suitable for the long-term treatment of CTD-ILD. We particularly like to use AZA in RA-ILD because this agent can help control both the synovitic and ILD components, and, when needed for more effective synovitis control, we combine AZA with a biologic DMARD.

### Mycophenolate Mofetil

MMF has become an increasingly popular treatment in CTD-ILD. The first series advocating MMF in CTD-ILD comprised 28 subjects and showed that MMF was well tolerated and associated with preservation of lung function among a diverse spectrum of CTD-ILD.[32] Several other small series have suggested a beneficial role of MMF for SSc-ILD.[32–34] The largest study of MMF use for CTD-ILD[35] included a heterogeneous cohort of 125 patients with CTD-ILD (44 SSc-ILD, 32 IIM-ILD, 18 RA-ILD), with a mean age of 60.4 ± 11.6 years; 42% were women and most were treated with MMF 3 g/d over a 3-year period. In this large and diverse CTD-ILD retrospective cohort, MMF treatment was associated with effective CS dose tapering (from a median of 20 mg/d to 5 mg/d of prednisone at 12 months from MMF initiation [$P$<.0001]). MMF was also associated with longitudinal improvements in FVC and DLco and was a well-tolerated therapy (~90% adherence rate).

In our experience, MMF is often an effective agent in the management of CTD-ILD. In addition, similar to AZA, MMF is well tolerated and can be safely combined with biologic DMARDs in CTD-ILD when needed to control extrathoracic disease manifestations (eg, synovitis).

### Calcineurin Antagonists

Several retrospective studies suggest beneficial roles of cyclosporine and tacrolimus in CTD-ILD. Harigai and colleagues[36] reported the use of cyclosporine in 48 patients with CTD-ILD (26 IIM, 7 SSc, 7 RA, 8 other CTDs). Cyclosporine was effective for 72.2% and 33.3% in acute cases versus 50.0% and 50.0% in chronic cases in the IIM-ILD and other CTD-ILD, respectively. A more recent study retrospectively reviewed 17 patients with antisynthetase syndrome–ILD who failed prednisone within 12 months of ILD onset and subsequently started cyclosporine.[37] At 2 years of follow-up, FVC increased from 65% to 76% of predicted and DLco from 55% to 63% of predicted. The results were substantially maintained, including at the last available follow-up (median follow-up time, 96 months). Tacrolimus can be an effective agent for the spectrum of CTD-ILD and, perhaps, in IIM-ILD in particular. In a retrospective study, 13 patients with both myositis and ILD[38] were treated with tacrolimus for a mean period of 51.2 months, showing maintained improvement in myositis, FVC, and DLco during 150 weeks of follow-up. Other observations show potential efficacy in refractory cases previously treated with combination therapies including CYC and cyclosporine[39–41] and addition of tacrolimus on conventional therapy (prednisolone, IV CYC, and/or cyclosporine) was shown to be associated with better survival.[42]

### Rituximab

Several recent reports suggest that RTX may be an effective agent for CTD-ILD. Keir and colleagues[43] reported 8 cases of CTD-ILD (5 IIM-ILD; median FVC, 45% of predicted; median DLco, 25% of predicted) in which RTX was used as rescue therapy. Six of these patients had serial pulmonary function tests (PFTs): before RTX infusion, all had decline in FVC and DLco, and after RTX infusion, a median DLco improvement of 22% ($P = .04$) and a median FVC improvement of 18% ($P = .03$) were noted. The same group recently reported their experience with RTX infusions in 50 cases of severe and refractory ILD; 33 of these cases had CTD-ILD (10 IIM, 8 SSc, 9 undifferentiated CTD), 4 required mechanical ventilation, DLco was 24.5% of predicted, and FVC was 44.0% of predicted.[44] In the CTD-ILD subgroup, 85% of the patients (most with IIM) were classified as responders. In the 6 to 12 months before RTX, a median decline in FVC of 13.3% and in DLco of 18.8% were noted compared with the 6 to 12 months after RTX therapy, in which an improvement of 8.9% of the FVC ($P<.01$) and a stabilization of the DLco ($P<.01$) were noted. Dodds and colleagues[45] also reported their retrospective experience of RTX use in 22 patients with severe refractory CTD-ILD as rescue therapy (5 RA, 7 IIM, 2 SLE, 2 SSc, 3 other CTDs). Nine patients showed radiographic stability or improvement, whereas 4 patients showed deterioration under RTX. In those patients in whom RTX prevented disease progression (n = 8), there was improvement in FVC (+2.5%; range, 0%–7%; $P = .08$) over an average period of 19 months.

There are several small studies of RTX in SSc-ILD. With secondary end points of PFT and thoracic HRCT scan, 15 patients with dcSSc, and FVC and DLco greater than or equal to 50% of predicted received the RA regimen. At 6 months, the FVC, the DLco, and the thoracic HRCT scan remained stable.[46] Daoussis and colleagues[47] reported the results of a small randomized controlled trial of 8 patients with SSc-ILD treated with the vasculitis protocol (375 mg/m$^2$ weekly for 4 weeks) and then again 6 months later compared with 6 subjects receiving standard treatment (including prednisone, MMF, CYC, and bosentan). At 1 year, the FVC in the RTX group increased by 10.3% (68.1% ± 19.7% to 75.6% ± 19.7%; $P = .0018$) compared with the control group (86.0% ± 19.6% to 81.7% ± 20.7%; $P = .23$) losing 5.0% ($P = .002$). The DLco also improved by 9.7% (52.3% ± 20.7% to 62.0% ± 23.2%; $P = .017$) compared with a decrease of 7.5% ($P = .023$) in the control group (65.3% ± 21.4% to 60.2% ± 23.7%; $P = .25$). Follow-up of the RTX-treated patients at 2 years from the first infusion showed stability for both FVC and DLco ($P<.0001$ for both values).[48]

Several case reports suggest that RTX may have a role in severe, refractory IIM-ILD.[49] A small retrospective series of 11 patients with antisynthetase syndrome–ILD were treated with RTX as a rescue therapy.[50] Comparing the 8 months' pretreatment data and the 7 months' posttreatment PFT data, 6 patients had an FVC improvement of greater than 10% and 3 had a DLco increase of greater than 15%. Three to 6 months following infusion, the thoracic HRCT scan showed a regression of the ground-glass opacities in 4 patients and progression in 1. In another study by Unger and colleagues,[51] 8 patients with IIM-ILD were treated with RTX. The baseline FVC of 74% ± 19% of predicted increased to 83% ± 21% of predicted at 7 months, 91% ± 21% of predicted at 12 months, and 108% ± 15% of predicted at 21 months following the initial cycle (4 of these patients received more than 1 RTX cycle). The DLco was not significantly improved at 6 months from the initial RTX cycle.

In addition, the results of 10 patients with RA-ILD (4 UIP, 6 NSIP, baseline FVC 68% [range, 47%–89%], baseline DLco, 48% [range, 28%–73%]) treated with RTX was recently reported.[52] Of the 7 subjects with data at baseline and 48 weeks, FVC and DLco worsened in 1 subject, stabilized in 4, and improved by greater than 10% in 2 (at 48 weeks, FVC 75% [range, 50%–102%] and DLco, 52% [range, 30%–75%]). Also, among 188 patients with RA-ILD in 16 centers across the United Kingdom during a 25-year period (65% UIP), 57 patients were treated with a biologic agent. No difference in all-cause or respiratory mortality was noted in patients treated with biologics versus other agents. However, there was a statistically significant difference in respiratory mortality between patients treated with anti-TNF (n = 30) versus RTX (n = 27) (15% vs 4%; $P = .04$) and in all-cause mortality in 31% of patients treated with anti-TNF versus 8% of patients treated with RTX ($P = .03$) in the UIP subgroup.[10]

The role of RTX for CTD-ILD remains to be defined. This agent may have a role in specific subsets of CTD-ILD, such as the antisynthetase syndrome and those cases in which lung biopsy suggests a role of B cells in the ILD pathogenesis. Further studies are needed to more precisely define its role in CTD-ILD.

### Future Directions in the Pharmacologic Treatment of Connective Tissue Disease–associated Interstitial Lung Disease

There have been several novel antifibrotic therapies studied in ILD but these have almost exclusively been limited to clinical trials for patients with IPF. The only antifibrotic agent studied in CTD-ILD was bosentan for SSc-ILD in the BUILD-2 trial,[53] which showed that bosentan is ineffective for the ILD in SSc. Recent studies of pirfenidone and nintedanib have shown a positive impact on disease progression in patients with IPF[54–56]; however, there are currently no data to support their use in CTD-ILD. There is an ongoing phase II study addressing safety and tolerability of pirfenidone for SSc-ILD (LOTUSS trial; NCT01933334).

## NONPHARMACOLOGIC STRATEGIES AND ADDRESSING COMORBIDITIES
### Cardiopulmonary Rehabilitation

Cardiopulmonary rehabilitation is an important adjunctive therapy for several chronic lung diseases, including ILD.[57] Although not formally studied in CTD-ILD, we find cardiopulmonary rehabilitation to be useful for both the ILD component as well as some of the extrathoracic disease components (eg, muscle strengthening).

### Oxygen Supplementation

Although not formally studied in CTD-ILD, we believe that the need for supplemental oxygen should be evaluated in all patients with ILD, to ensure absence of hypoxia while at rest, with exercise, and with sleep. A few studies in ILD show improvement of exercise capacity with oxygen supplementation but data on patient-related outcomes and survival are lacking.[58] In addition, given how commonly CSs are used, consideration for obstructive sleep apnea detection is warranted.

### Gastroesophageal Reflux Disease and Aspiration

Gastroesophageal reflux disease (GERD) and esophageal dysmotility are common troublesome medical conditions frequently encountered in patients with CTD-ILD,[59,60] and can often be difficult to treat. General measures such as avoidance of specific foods that decrease the lower esophageal sphincter tone, eating multiple smaller portions throughout the day, avoiding eating or drinking before going to bed, and elevating the head of the bed are important to implement.[61] Proton pump inhibitor and H2-receptor antagonist therapies are commonly required, sometimes at higher dosage and often in combination. Promotility agents (eg, domperidone) are sometimes needed as well. In addition, fundoplication is sometimes attempted for recurrent aspiration pneumonia or in anticipation of lung transplantation, but has a potential to worsen the esophageal dysmotility present in patients with CTD.[62]

### Pulmonary Hypertension

Patients with ILD are at an increased risk of secondary pulmonary hypertension (PH) partly because of chronic hypoxia.[63] In addition, patients with SSc, SLE, and mixed CTD are at risk for a primary vasculopathy resulting in pulmonary arterial hypertension.[64] In our opinion, periodic screening with echocardiography should be considered in all patients with CTD-ILD, even if there are limitations to this procedure in advanced lung disease.[65] In patients with SSc-ILD, Steen and Medsger[66] showed that an FVC/DLco ratio greater than 1.6 suggests concomitant PH. Also, increases in the serum brain natriuretic peptide level also suggest the presence of PH[67] but can be normal with PH proved by right-heart catheterization (RHC).[68] Any suspicion of PH on noninvasive assessment should be followed by a definitive evaluation with RHC. There are no controlled data to treat PH in patients with concomitant ILD and PH, even in SSc. In practice, immunosuppressive regimens for ILD with PH-targeted therapies are often combined based on anecdotal evidence[69,70] and recent data suggest that these approaches may be ineffective.[71]

### Acute Interstitial Lung Disease Exacerbations

Patients with CTD-ILD are at risk for disease exacerbations,[72] and these are typically associated with a poor outcome.[73,74] When a patient with CTD-ILD develops acute or subacute worsening breathlessness or cough, ILD exacerbation is a concern, and comprehensive evaluation is indicated to exclude more common entities such as respiratory infection, thromboembolism, or acute cardiovascular events. Such evaluation may require a multidisciplinary approach. Drug-induced pneumonitis associated with immunosuppressive agents (such as CYC-associated pneumonitis) cannot be ignored as a possibility. Management of acute exacerbation, particularly in CTD-ILD, lacks controlled data. Our approach is to use high-dose CS as a first-line agent, followed by consideration of altering or intensifying the secondary immunosuppressive therapies. Some patients also need mechanical ventilation support and mixed results have been obtained from emergent lung transplantation in this clinical scenario.[75]

### Smoking Cessation

Smoking cessation is a fundamental component of treating any chronic lung disease and CTD-ILD is no different because these patients can have multiple pathophysiologic processes to their ILD.

## Immunizations

Considering the presence of intrinsic lung disease and that many patients with CTD have inherent immunodeficiency and are on chronic immunosuppressive treatment, basic infection prevention practices should be taught and emphasized, and appropriate vaccinations should be administered (**Table 1**).[76–78] Because of its higher incidence in CTDs in general,[79] herpes zoster vaccine, which is safe in this population,[80] should be considered in all patients with CTD independently of age and prior episode status.[76]

## Pneumocystis Prophylaxis

*Pneumocystis jiroveci* pneumonia (PjP) is an atypical infection with potentially severe consequences in CTD-ILD.[81,82] It may be more difficult to diagnose and is associated with a worse prognosis in the rheumatologic population compared with the human immunodeficiency virus/AIDS population.[83] PjP prophylaxis is recommended when 2 immunosuppressive therapies (including CS $\geq$ 20 mg/d of prednisone equivalent[84]) are used. Some practitioners also recommend it when using CS at greater than or

**Table 1**
**Suggested immunization schedule for individuals with CTD-ILD**

| Vaccines | Schedule and Particularities |
|---|---|
| Influenza vaccine (intramuscular) | Annually unless contraindicated |
| Pneumococcal vaccine<br>• PCV13 vaccine<br>• PPSV23 vaccine | If never vaccinated:<br>• PCV13 first followed by PPSV23 8 wk later<br>• PPSV23 each 5 y after<br>If previously vaccinated with PPSV23:<br>• PCV13 should be administered no sooner than 1 y after PPSV23<br>• PPSV23 each 5 y after (and at least 8 wk after PCV13 if recent) |
| Other inactivated vaccines (eg, TDaP, HPV, HBV) | Usual recommended schedule<br>Ideally before starting immunosuppressive therapy<br>Acceptable under DMARDs and biologics, except for RTX, for which should be given 4 wk before or 6 mo after infusion |
| Live attenuated vaccines (eg, BCG, nasal/oral influenza, MMR) | Consult specialist<br>Ideally 4 wk before immunosuppression and at least 5 half-lives after therapy discontinuation |
| Herpes zoster vaccine (live attenuated vaccine) | Independent of age and prior episode status<br>Ideally before starting immunosuppressive therapy; can be given with CS at <20 mg/d of prednisone equivalent or $\geq$20 mg/d if used for <2 wk or AZA<3 mg/kg/d<br>Other immunosuppressive agents (like MMF) or higher doses of the agents mentioned earlier should be stopped for 4 wk before herpes zoster vaccine administration<br>Seek expert advice before administration on continued immunosuppressive therapy |

*Abbreviations:* BCG, bacillus Calmette-Guérin; HBV, hepatitis B virus; HPV, human papilloma virus; MMF, mycophenolate mofetil; MMR, measles-mumps-rubella; PCV13, pneumococcal 13-valent conjugate; PPSV23, pneumococcal polysaccharide; TDaP, diphtheria-tetanus-acellular pertussis.
*Data from* Refs.[76–78]

equal to 20 mg/d of prednisone equivalent alone for any sustained period of time or CYC in single therapy. In addition, PjP is a possible diagnosis in any patient with CTD with new respiratory deterioration and lung infiltrates.

## Bone Health Measures

Bone health aspects in patients with CTD-ILD should be addressed, integrating longitudinal bone densitometry follow-up, good bone habits (diet, exercise, alcohol and tobacco avoidance, and so forth), adequate intakes of calcium and vitamin D, and usage of bone antiresorptive agent prophylactically as indicated. It is important to keep in mind that even low doses of CS ($\leq$5 mg daily of prednisone equivalent) are associated with an increased fracture risk[85] and that guidelines about who should be prophylactically treated have been published.[86]

## Lung Transplantation

Lung transplantation is a last resort in the management of CTD-ILD. Careful selection of suitable patients for lung transplantation is a complex and tedious process and thorough evaluations are needed, often sooner than later to avoid gaps in care. Notable manifestations that can complicate or preclude transplantation include concurrent PH; heart failure; renal disease; thromboembolic disease; chest wall skin thickening; and, in particular, severe GERD with dysmotility or aspiration. Furthermore, the overall activity of the extrathoracic CTD manifestations needs to be considered as well as the degree of associated functional impairment or disability attributable to the extrathoracic features. Mortality in transplanted patients with SSc-ILD is comparable with that of IPF at 2 years (38% in SSc vs 33% in IPF).[87] Another study showed no survival difference at 1 year between patients with SSc and IPF but rates of acute graft rejection were significantly increased for the SSc group compared with the IPF group (hazard ratio, 2.91; $P$<.007), contrary to other adverse effects that were similar in occurence.[88]

## FUTURE CONSIDERATIONS/SUMMARY

The intersection of the CTDs and the ILDs is complex. Although often considered as a single entity, CTD-ILD reflects a heterogeneous spectrum of diverse CTDs and a variety of patterns of IP. Pharmacologic intervention with immunosuppression is the mainstay of therapy for all forms of CTD-ILD, but should be reserved only for those that show clinically significant and/or progressive disease. The management of CTD-ILD is not yet evidence based and there is an urgent need for controlled trials across the spectrum of CTD-ILD. Nonpharmacologic management strategies (eg, supplemental oxygen and cardiopulmonary rehabilitation) and addressing comorbidities or aggravating factors (eg, GERD, aspiration, bone health, PH, PjP prophylaxis) should be part of a comprehensive treatment plan for individuals with CTD-ILD.

## REFERENCES

1. Roubille C, Haraoui B. Interstitial lung diseases induced or exacerbated by DMARDS and biologic agents in rheumatoid arthritis: a systematic literature review. Semin Arthritis Rheum 2014;43(5):613–26.
2. Kremer JM, Alarcon GS, Weinblatt ME, et al. Clinical, laboratory, radiographic, and histopathologic features of methotrexate-associated lung injury in patients with rheumatoid arthritis: a multicenter study with literature review. Arthritis Rheum 1997;40(10):1829–37.

3. Golden MR, Katz RS, Balk RA, et al. The relationship of preexisting lung disease to the development of methotrexate pneumonitis in patients with rheumatoid arthritis. J Rheumatol 1995;22(6):1043–7.

4. Taylor PC, Feldmann M. Anti-TNF biologic agents: still the therapy of choice for rheumatoid arthritis. Nat Rev Rheumatol 2009;5(10):578–82.

5. Karampetsou MP, Liossis SN, Sfikakis PP. TNF-alpha antagonists beyond approved indications: stories of success and prospects for the future. QJM 2010;103(12):917–28.

6. Dixon WG, Hyrich KL, Watson KD, et al. Influence of anti-TNF therapy on mortality in patients with rheumatoid arthritis-associated interstitial lung disease: results from the British Society for Rheumatology Biologics Register. Ann Rheum Dis 2010;69(6):1086–91.

7. Takeuchi T, Tatsuki Y, Nogami Y, et al. Postmarketing surveillance of the safety profile of infliximab in 5000 Japanese patients with rheumatoid arthritis. Ann Rheum Dis 2008;67(2):189–94.

8. Koike T, Harigai M, Inokuma S, et al. Postmarketing surveillance of the safety and effectiveness of etanercept in Japan. J Rheumatol 2009;36(5):898–906.

9. Panopoulos ST, Sfikakis PP. Biological treatments and connective tissue disease associated interstitial lung disease. Curr Opin Pulm Med 2011;17(5):362–7.

10. Palmer E, Kelly C, Nisar M, et al. Rheumatoid-arthritis-related interstitial lung disease: association between biologic therapy and survival. Rheumatology (Oxford) 2014;53(9):1676–82.

11. Nakashita T, Ando K, Kaneko N, et al. Potential risk of TNF inhibitors on the progression of interstitial lung disease in patients with rheumatoid arthritis. BMJ Open 2014;4(8):e005615.

12. Ando K, Motojima S, Doi T, et al. Effect of glucocorticoid monotherapy on pulmonary function and survival in Japanese patients with scleroderma-related interstitial lung disease. Respir Investig 2013;51(2):69–75.

13. Horai Y, Isomoto E, Koga T, et al. Early diagnosis and treatment for remission of clinically amyopathic dermatomyositis complicated by rapid progress interstitial lung disease: a report of two cases. Mod Rheumatol 2013;23(1):190–4.

14. Steen VD, Medsger TA Jr. Case-control study of corticosteroids and other drugs that either precipitate or protect from the development of scleroderma renal crisis. Arthritis Rheum 1998;41(9):1613–9.

15. Collard HR, Ryu JH, Douglas WW, et al. Combined corticosteroid and cyclophosphamide therapy does not alter survival in idiopathic pulmonary fibrosis. Chest 2004;125(6):2169–74.

16. Raghu G, Anstrom KJ, King TE Jr, et al. Prednisone, azathioprine, and N-acetyl-cysteine for pulmonary fibrosis. N Engl J Med 2012;366(21):1968–77.

17. Silver RM, Warrick JH, Kinsella MB, et al. Cyclophosphamide and low-dose prednisone therapy in patients with systemic sclerosis (scleroderma) with interstitial lung disease. J Rheumatol 1993;20(5):838–44.

18. Schnabel A, Reuter M, Gross WL. Intravenous pulse cyclophosphamide in the treatment of interstitial lung disease due to collagen vascular diseases. Arthritis Rheum 1998;41(7):1215–20.

19. Akesson A, Scheja A, Lundin A, et al. Improved pulmonary function in systemic sclerosis after treatment with cyclophosphamide. Arthritis Rheum 1994;37(5):729–35.

20. White B, Moore WC, Wigley FM, et al. Cyclophosphamide is associated with pulmonary function and survival benefit in patients with scleroderma and alveolitis. Ann Intern Med 2000;132(12):947–54.

21. Steen VD, Lanz JK Jr, Conte C, et al. Therapy for severe interstitial lung disease in systemic sclerosis. A retrospective study. Arthritis Rheum 1994;37(9):1290–6.
22. Tashkin DP, Elashoff R, Clements PJ, et al. Cyclophosphamide versus placebo in scleroderma lung disease. N Engl J Med 2006;354(25):2655–66.
23. Tashkin DP, Elashoff R, Clements PJ, et al. Effects of 1-year treatment with cyclophosphamide on outcomes at 2 years in scleroderma lung disease. Am J Respir Crit Care Med 2007;176(10):1026–34.
24. Roth MD, Tseng CH, Clements PJ, et al. Predicting treatment outcomes and responder subsets in scleroderma-related interstitial lung disease. Arthritis Rheum 2011;63(9):2797–808.
25. Hoyles RK, Ellis RW, Wellsbury J, et al. A multicenter, prospective, randomized, double-blind, placebo-controlled trial of corticosteroids and intravenous cyclophosphamide followed by oral azathioprine for the treatment of pulmonary fibrosis in scleroderma. Arthritis Rheum 2006;54(12):3962–70.
26. Mira-Avendano IC, Parambil JG, Yadav R, et al. A retrospective review of clinical features and treatment outcomes in steroid-resistant interstitial lung disease from polymyositis/dermatomyositis. Respir Med 2013;107(6):890–6.
27. Yamasaki Y, Yamada H, Yamasaki M, et al. Intravenous cyclophosphamide therapy for progressive interstitial pneumonia in patients with polymyositis/dermatomyositis. Rheumatology (Oxford) 2007;46(1):124–30.
28. Berezne A, Ranque B, Valeyre D, et al. Therapeutic strategy combining intravenous cyclophosphamide followed by oral azathioprine to treat worsening interstitial lung disease associated with systemic sclerosis: a retrospective multicenter open-label study. J Rheumatol 2008;35(6):1064–72.
29. Dheda K, Lalloo UG, Cassim B, et al. Experience with azathioprine in systemic sclerosis associated with interstitial lung disease. Clin Rheumatol 2004;23(4):306–9.
30. Poormoghim H, Rezaei N, Sheidaie Z, et al. Systemic sclerosis: comparison of efficacy of oral cyclophosphamide and azathioprine on skin score and pulmonary involvement-a retrospective study. Rheumatol Int 2014;34(12):1691–9.
31. Deheinzelin D, Capelozzi VL, Kairalla RA, et al. Interstitial lung disease in primary Sjogren's syndrome. Clinical-pathological evaluation and response to treatment. Am J Respir Crit Care Med 1996;154(3 Pt 1):794–9.
32. Swigris JJ, Olson AL, Fischer A, et al. Mycophenolate mofetil is safe, well tolerated, and preserves lung function in patients with connective tissue disease-related interstitial lung disease. Chest 2006;130(1):30–6.
33. Gerbino AJ, Goss CH, Molitor JA. Effect of mycophenolate mofetil on pulmonary function in scleroderma-associated interstitial lung disease. Chest 2008;133(2):455–60.
34. Liossis SN, Bounas A, Andonopoulos AP. Mycophenolate mofetil as first-line treatment improves clinically evident early scleroderma lung disease. Rheumatology (Oxford) 2006;45(8):1005–8.
35. Fischer A, Brown KK, Du Bois RM, et al. Mycophenolate mofetil improves lung function in connective tissue disease-associated interstitial lung disease. J Rheumatol 2013;40(5):640–6.
36. Harigai M, Hara M, Kamatani N, et al. Nation-wide survey for the treatment with cyclosporin A of interstitial pneumonia associated with collagen diseases. Ryumachi 1999;39(6):819–28.
37. Cavagna L, Caporali R, Abdi-Ali L, et al. Cyclosporine in anti-Jo1-positive patients with corticosteroid-refractory interstitial lung disease. J Rheumatol 2013;40(4):484–92.

38. Wilkes MR, Sereika SM, Fertig N, et al. Treatment of antisynthetase-associated interstitial lung disease with tacrolimus. Arthritis Rheum 2005;52(8):2439–46.
39. Takada K, Nagasaka K, Miyasaka N. Polymyositis/dermatomyositis and interstitial lung disease: a new therapeutic approach with T-cell-specific immunosuppressants. Autoimmunity 2005;38(5):383–92.
40. Ochi S, Nanki T, Takada K, et al. Favorable outcomes with tacrolimus in two patients with refractory interstitial lung disease associated with polymyositis/dermatomyositis. Clin Exp Rheumatol 2005;23(5):707–10.
41. Oddis CV, Sciurba FC, Elmagd KA, et al. Tacrolimus in refractory polymyositis with interstitial lung disease. Lancet 1999;353(9166):1762–3.
42. Kurita T, Yasuda S, Oba K, et al. The efficacy of tacrolimus in patients with interstitial lung diseases complicated with polymyositis or dermatomyositis. Rheumatology (Oxford) 2015;54:39–44.
43. Keir GJ, Maher TM, Hansell DM, et al. Severe interstitial lung disease in connective tissue disease: rituximab as rescue therapy. Eur Respir J 2012; 40(3):641–8.
44. Keir GJ, Maher TM, Ming D, et al. Rituximab in severe, treatment-refractory interstitial lung disease. Respirology 2014;19:353–9.
45. Dodds NL, Lamb H, Mayers L, et al. Rituximab therapy for refractory interstitial lung disease unresponsive to conventional immunosuppression: a case series. Am J Respir Crit Care Med 2014;189:A1451.
46. Lafyatis R, Kissin E, York M, et al. B cell depletion with rituximab in patients with diffuse cutaneous systemic sclerosis. Arthritis Rheum 2009;60(2):578–83.
47. Daoussis D, Liossis SN, Tsamandas AC, et al. Experience with rituximab in scleroderma: results from a 1-year, proof-of-principle study. Rheumatology (Oxford) 2010;49(2):271–80.
48. Daoussis D, Liossis SN, Tsamandas AC, et al. Effect of long-term treatment with rituximab on pulmonary function and skin fibrosis in patients with diffuse systemic sclerosis. Clin Exp Rheumatol 2012;30(2 Suppl 71):S17–22.
49. Vandenbroucke E, Grutters JC, Altenburg J, et al. Rituximab in life threatening antisynthetase syndrome. Rheumatol Int 2009;29(12):1499–502.
50. Sem M, Molberg O, Lund MB, et al. Rituximab treatment of the anti-synthetase syndrome: a retrospective case series. Rheumatology (Oxford) 2009;48(8): 968–71.
51. Unger L, Kampf S, Luthke K, et al. Rituximab therapy in patients with refractory dermatomyositis or polymyositis: differential effects in a real-life population. Rheumatology (Oxford) 2014;53(9):1630–8.
52. Matteson E, Bongartz T, Ryu J, et al. Open-label, pilot study of the safety and clinical effects of rituximab in patients with rheumatoid arthritis-associated interstitial pneumonia. Open J Rheumatol Autoimmune Dis 2012;2(3):53–8.
53. Seibold JR, Denton CP, Furst DE, et al. Randomized, prospective, placebo-controlled trial of bosentan in interstitial lung disease secondary to systemic sclerosis. Arthritis Rheum 2010;62(7):2101–8.
54. Noble PW, Albera C, Bradford WZ, et al. Pirfenidone in patients with idiopathic pulmonary fibrosis (CAPACITY): two randomised trials. Lancet 2011;377(9779): 1760–9.
55. King TE Jr, Bradford WZ, Castro-Bernardini S, et al. A phase 3 trial of pirfenidone in patients with idiopathic pulmonary fibrosis. N Engl J Med 2014;370(22): 2083–92.
56. Richeldi L, du Bois RM, Raghu G, et al. Efficacy and safety of nintedanib in idiopathic pulmonary fibrosis. N Engl J Med 2014;370(22):2071–82.

57. Johnson-Warrington V, Williams J, Bankart J, et al. Pulmonary rehabilitation and interstitial lung disease: aiding the referral decision. J Cardiopulm Rehabil Prev 2013;33(3):189–95.

58. Visca D, Montgomery A, de Lauretis A, et al. Ambulatory oxygen in interstitial lung disease. Eur Respir J 2011;38(4):987–90.

59. Ntoumazios SK, Voulgari PV, Potsis K, et al. Esophageal involvement in scleroderma: gastroesophageal reflux, the common problem. Semin Arthritis Rheum 2006;36(3):173–81.

60. Miura Y, Fukuda K, Maeda T, et al. Gastroesophageal reflux disease in patients with rheumatoid arthritis. Mod Rheumatol 2014;24(2):291–5.

61. Bredenoord AJ, Pandolfino JE, Smout AJ. Gastro-oesophageal reflux disease. Lancet 2013;381(9881):1933–42.

62. Weinstein WM, Kadell BM. The gastrointestinal tract in systemic sclerosis. In: Clements PJ, Furst DE, editors. Systemic sclerosis, vol. xvii, 2nd edition. Philadelphia: Lippincott Williams & Wilkins; 2004. p. 293–308.

63. Nathan SD, Hassoun PM. Pulmonary hypertension due to lung disease and/or hypoxia. Clin Chest Med 2013;34(4):695–705.

64. Ahmed S, Palevsky HI. Pulmonary arterial hypertension related to connective tissue disease: a review. Rheum Dis Clin North Am 2014;40(1):103–24.

65. Arcasoy SM, Christie JD, Ferrari VA, et al. Echocardiographic assessment of pulmonary hypertension in patients with advanced lung disease. Am J Respir Crit Care Med 2003;167(5):735–40.

66. Steen V, Medsger TA Jr. Predictors of isolated pulmonary hypertension in patients with systemic sclerosis and limited cutaneous involvement. Arthritis Rheum 2003; 48(2):516–22.

67. Allanore Y, Borderie D, Avouac J, et al. High N-terminal pro-brain natriuretic peptide levels and low diffusing capacity for carbon monoxide as independent predictors of the occurrence of precapillary pulmonary arterial hypertension in patients with systemic sclerosis. Arthritis Rheum 2008;58(1):284–91.

68. Miller L, Chartrand S, Koenig M, et al. Left heart disease: a frequent cause of early pulmonary hypertension in systemic sclerosis, unrelated to elevated NT-proBNP levels or overt cardiac fibrosis but associated with increased levels of MR-proANP and MR-proADM: retrospective analysis of a French Canadian cohort. Scand J Rheumatol 2014;43(4):314–23.

69. Olschewski H, Ghofrani HA, Walmrath D, et al. Inhaled prostacyclin and iloprost in severe pulmonary hypertension secondary to lung fibrosis. Am J Respir Crit Care Med 1999;160(2):600–7.

70. Shapiro S. Management of pulmonary hypertension resulting from interstitial lung disease. Curr Opin Pulm Med 2003;9(5):426–30.

71. Corte TJ, Keir GJ, Dimopoulos K, et al. Bosentan in pulmonary hypertension associated with fibrotic idiopathic interstitial pneumonia. Am J Respir Crit Care Med 2014;190(2):208–17.

72. Solomon JJ, Fischer A. Connective tissue disease-associated interstitial lung disease: a focused review. J Intensive Care Med 2013. [Epub ahead of print].

73. Suda T, Kaida Y, Nakamura Y, et al. Acute exacerbation of interstitial pneumonia associated with collagen vascular diseases. Respir Med 2009;103(6):846–53.

74. Tachikawa R, Tomii K, Ueda H, et al. Clinical features and outcome of acute exacerbation of interstitial pneumonia: collagen vascular diseases-related versus idiopathic. Respiration 2012;83(1):20–7.

75. Boussaud V, Mal H, Trinquart L, et al. One-year experience with high-emergency lung transplantation in France. Transplantation 2012;93(10):1058–63.

76. Bridges CB, Coyne-Beasley T. Advisory committee on immunization practices recommended immunization schedule for adults aged 19 years or older: United States, 2014. Ann Intern Med 2014;160(3):190.

77. Bombardier C, Hazlewood GS, Akhavan P, et al. Canadian Rheumatology Association recommendations for the pharmacological management of rheumatoid arthritis with traditional and biologic disease-modifying antirheumatic drugs: part II safety. J Rheumatol 2012;39(8):1583–602.

78. van Assen S, Agmon-Levin N, Elkayam O, et al. EULAR recommendations for vaccination in adult patients with autoimmune inflammatory rheumatic diseases. Ann Rheum Dis 2011;70(3):414–22.

79. Veetil BM, Myasoedova E, Matteson EL, et al. Incidence and time trends of herpes zoster in rheumatoid arthritis: a population-based cohort study. Arthritis Care Res 2013;65(6):854–61.

80. Zhang J, Delzell E, Xie F, et al. The use, safety, and effectiveness of herpes zoster vaccination in individuals with inflammatory and autoimmune diseases: a longitudinal observational study. Arthritis Res Ther 2011;13(5):R174.

81. Sepkowitz KA. Opportunistic infections in patients with and patients without acquired immunodeficiency syndrome. Clin Infect Dis 2002;34(8):1098–107.

82. Iikuni N, Kitahama M, Ohta S, et al. Evaluation of *Pneumocystis* pneumonia infection risk factors in patients with connective tissue disease. Mod Rheumatol 2006; 16(5):282–8.

83. Sowden E, Carmichael AJ. Autoimmune inflammatory disorders, systemic corticosteroids and pneumocystis pneumonia: a strategy for prevention. BMC Infect Dis 2004;4:42.

84. Vananuvat P, Suwannalai P, Sungkanuparph S, et al. Primary prophylaxis for *Pneumocystis jirovecii* pneumonia in patients with connective tissue diseases. Semin Arthritis Rheum 2011;41(3):497–502.

85. Van Staa TP, Leufkens HG, Abenhaim L, et al. Use of oral corticosteroids and risk of fractures. June, 2000. J Bone Miner Res 2005;20(8):1487–94 [discussion: 1486].

86. Grossman JM, Gordon R, Ranganath VK, et al. American College of Rheumatology 2010 recommendations for the prevention and treatment of glucocorticoid-induced osteoporosis. Arthritis Care Res 2010;62(11):1515–26.

87. Schachna L, Medsger TA Jr, Dauber JH, et al. Lung transplantation in scleroderma compared with idiopathic pulmonary fibrosis and idiopathic pulmonary arterial hypertension. Arthritis Rheum 2006;54(12):3954–61.

88. Saggar R, Khanna D, Furst DE, et al. Systemic sclerosis and bilateral lung transplantation: a single centre experience. Eur Respir J 2010;36(4):893–900.

# Connective Tissue Disease–Associated Pulmonary Arterial Hypertension

 CrossMark

Yon K. Sung, MD[a], Lorinda Chung, MD, MS[b,c],*

## KEYWORDS

- Pulmonary hypertension • Pulmonary arterial hypertension
- Connective tissue disease • Systemic sclerosis • Systemic lupus erythematosus
- Mixed connective tissue disease

## KEY POINTS

- Systemic sclerosis is the most common underlying disease associated with connective tissue disease–associated pulmonary arterial hypertension (CTD-PAH), and has the poorest prognosis.
- Patients with suspected PAH should undergo a complete evaluation, including right heart catheterization (RHC) and testing to rule out other possible causes of pulmonary hypertension.
- Patients with RHC-confirmed PAH should be treated with PAH-specific therapies. However, the role of immunosuppression for the treatment of CTD-PAH is unclear.
- The development of robust screening algorithms may lead to earlier diagnosis and improved survival in systemic sclerosis-PAH.

## INTRODUCTION

Pulmonary hypertension (PH) is a disease that is strictly defined by having a resting mean pulmonary artery pressure (mPAP) of 25 mm Hg or greater as measured by right heart catheterization (RHC).[1] The causes of PH are diverse, but regardless of the cause, chronic elevation of pulmonary arterial pressures can lead to right ventricular

Disclosure: Y.K. Sung has received research support from Actelion. L. Chung has received research support funding from Gilead, United Therapeutics, Pfizer, and Actelion and has served on the Advisory Board for Gilead (<$10,000 per year).
a Division of Pulmonary and Critical Care Medicine, Vera Moulton Wall Center for Pulmonary Vascular Disease, Stanford University School of Medicine, 300 Pasteur Drive, Stanford, CA 94305, USA; b Division of Rheumatology and Immunology, Stanford University School of Medicine, 300 Pasteur Drive, Stanford, CA 94305, USA; c Division of Rheumatology, VA Palo Alto Health Care System, 3801 Miranda Avenue, Palo Alto, CA 94304, USA
* Corresponding author. VA Palo Alto Health Care System, 3801 Miranda Avenue, Palo Alto, CA 94304.
E-mail address: shauwei@stanford.edu

strain, dilatation, dysfunction, and ultimately right heart failure. Historically, PH was classified as either primary or secondary PH. However, it was recognized that this classification scheme was insufficient for distinguishing between different types of PH. At the second World Symposium on PH in 1998, the causes of PH were categorized into 5 groups: group 1, pulmonary arterial hypertension (PAH); group 2, PH secondary to left heart disease; group 3, PH owing to chronic lung disease and/or hypoxia; group 4, chronic thromboembolic PH; and group 5, PH owing to unclear multifactorial mechanisms.[2] Over the years, the classification scheme has been updated to reflect the growing understanding of the pathophysiology of different types of PH (**Box 1**).

PAH (previously primary PH) is a subset of PH that is characterized by remodeling of the small to medium sized pulmonary arterioles. It is defined as a mPAP of 25 mm Hg or greater, a pulmonary artery wedge pressure of 15 mm Hg or less, and a pulmonary vascular resistance of 3 or more Wood units, as measured by RHC.[1] Pathologically, it is characterized by eccentric and obliterative thickening of the intima and media, which are composed of mainly smooth muscle cells and myofibroblasts. The hallmark of PAH is the plexiform lesion, a disorganized growth of endothelial cells that form false channels.[3] Before the development of PAH-specific therapies, the prognosis of PAH was poor with a 1-year survival of 69% and a 5-year survival of 38%.[4]

It is well-known that patients with connective tissue diseases (CTD) are at increased risk for developing group 1 PAH. As demonstrated in large cohort studies, the CTD that is most commonly associated with PAH is systemic sclerosis (SSc).[5,6] Other associated CTDs are systemic lupus erythematosus (SLE), mixed CTD (MCTD), and less commonly, inflammatory myopathies (polymyositis [PM] and dermatomyositis), primary Sjogren's syndrome (pSS), rheumatoid arthritis (RA), and undifferentiated CTD.

As a group, the survival of patients with CTD-PAH is poorer compared with patients with other types of PAH. With increasing awareness of the morbidity and mortality associated with PAH in CTDs, there have been an increasing number of studies examining the burden of disease, pathophysiology, and risk factors associated with developing PAH in CTDs. Furthermore, because SSc is the most common CTD associated with PAH, recent studies have investigated screening methods for early detection of PAH in SSc with the hopes of decreasing morbidity and improving survival.

In this review, we summarize the current understanding of the epidemiology, pathophysiology, and known risk factors for CTD-PAH. Clinical presentation, evaluation, treatment, and prognosis are also reviewed. Although the focus of this review will be on group 1 PAH, it should be noted that patients with CTD are also at risk for developing other forms of PH. In particular, patients with CTD often have interstitial lung disease (ILD) and thus may have group 3 PH. Left heart dysfunction is also common in CTD, especially in SSc, so group 2 PH should be considered. Also, although a rare entity, pulmonary venoocclusive disease can be seen in patients with CTD. It is important to distinguish between these groups because the categorization has implications for prognosis and treatment.

## EPIDEMIOLOGY OF CONNECTIVE TISSUE DISEASE–ASSOCIATED PULMONARY ARTERIAL HYPERTENSION

Much of the data on the epidemiology of PAH has been obtained through multicenter national and international registries. Registries that have included patients with CTD-PAH include the French, US REVEAL (Registry to Evaluate Early and Long-Term PAH Disease Management), US Pulmonary Hypertension Connection Registry, Spanish, new Chinese, and COMPERA (European). In these registries, the percentage of PAH patients with CTD-PAH ranges from 15% to 30%.[7] As stated, the majority of patients

---

**Box 1**
**World Health Organization classification of PH**

1. PAH

   1.1 Idiopathic PAH

   1.2 Heritable PAH

      1.2.1 BMPR2

      1.2.2 ALK-1, ENG, SMAD9, CAV1, KCNK3

   1.3 Drug and toxin induced

   1.4 Associated with

      1.4.1 Connective tissue disease

      1.4.2 Human immunodeficiency virus

      1.4.3 Portal hypertension

      1.4.4 Congenital heart disease

      1.4.5 Schistosomiasis

1'. Pulmonary venoocclusive disease and/or pulmonary capillary hemangiomatosis

1". Persistent PH of the newborn (PPHN)

2. PH owing to left heart disease

   2.1 Left ventricular systolic dysfunction

   2.2 Left ventricular diastolic dysfunction

   2.3 Valvular disease

   2.4 Congenital/acquired left heart inflow/outflow tract obstruction and congenital cardiomyopathies

3. PH owing to lung disease and/or hypoxia

   3.1 Chronic obstructive pulmonary disease

   3.2 Interstitial lung disease

   3.3 Other pulmonary diseases with mixed restrictive and obstructive patterns

   3.4 Sleep-disordered breathing

   3.5 Alveolar hypoventilation disorders

   3.6 Chronic exposure to high altitude

   3.7 Developmental lung diseases

4. Chronic thromboembolic PH (CTEPH)

5. PH with unclear multifactorial mechanisms

   5.1 Hematologic disorders: chronic hemolytic anemia, myeloproliferative disorders, splenectomy

   5.2 Systemic disorders: sarcoidosis, pulmonary histiocytosis, lymphangioleiomyomatosis

   5.3 Metabolic disorders: glycogen storage disorders, Gaucher disease, thyroid disorders

   5.4 Others: tumoral obstruction, fibrosing mediastinitis, chronic renal failure, segmental PH

*Abbreviations:* PAH, pulmonary arterial hypertension; PH, pulmonary hypertension.
*From* Simonneau G, Gatzoulis MA, Adatia I, et al. Updated clinical classification of pulmonary hypertension. J Am Coll Cardiol 2013;62:D36; with permission.

with CTD-PAH have SSc. In the REVEAL registry, SSc accounted for 62.3% of CTD-PAH patients and a study of 429 CTD-PAH patients from a single center in the UK found that SSc accounted for 74% of the patients.[6] In an Australian cohort, 94.9% of CTD-PAH had SSc.[8] SLE is the next most common diagnosis, with 17.2% of CTD-PAH patients in the REVEAL registry and 8% of the UK cohort. MCTD accounted for 8% of CTD-PAH patients in REVEAL and the UK cohort. Interestingly, recent data suggest that this distribution may be unique to Western populations. In a cohort of 129 Chinese CTD-PAH patients, SSc only accounted for 6% of cases, whereas the majority was attributable to SLE at 49%.[9] A study of 321 Korean patients had a similar trend, with 35.3% of CTD-PAH patients attributable to SLE whereas 28.3% were secondary to SSc, although this study was limited by a low number of cases confirmed by RHC (**Table 1**).[10]

A number of studies have examined the prevalence of PAH in specific CTDs. In SSc patients, some larger studies have reported data with RHC confirmed PAH. However, few studies have examined the prevalence of PAH in non-SSc patients and the majority of these studies are based on elevations in right ventricular systolic pressure (RVSP) or pulmonary artery systolic pressure (PASP) on echocardiography alone without confirmation of the diagnosis with RHC. It is well-known that an elevated RVSP or PASP measurement on echocardiography is neither a sensitive nor specific test for the detection of PAH. A recent systematic review of the literature examined the accuracy of PASP on echocardiogram compared with PASP on RHC. These authors found that the correlation coefficient of PASP on echocardiogram compared with RHC was high at 0.84 for patients with left heart disease, but was much lower (0.58) for patients with right heart disease.[11] Moreover, the authors calculated that the difference between the echocardiographic and RHC measure differed by greater than 10 mm Hg in 37.6% of cases.[11] Another limitation of some of these prevalence studies is that

**Table 1**
**Distribution of diagnoses in CTD-PAH**

|  | UK Cohort,[6] No. of Patients (%) | US REVEAL Cohort,[5] No. of Patients (%) | Chinese Cohort,[9] No. of Patients (%) | Korean Registry,[10,a] No. of Patients (%) |
|---|---|---|---|---|
| SSc | 315 (74) | 399 (62.3)[b] | 8 (6) | 91 (28.3) |
| SLE | 35 (8) | 110 (17.2) | 62 (49) | 115 (35.3) |
| MCTD | 36 (8) | 52 (8.1) | (9) | 19 (5.9) |
| RA | 13 (3) | 28 (4.4) | (3) | 25 (7.8) |
| DM/PM | 18 (3) | 6 (0.9) | — | 14 (4.4) |
| pSS | 3 (1) | 13 (2.0) | (16) | — |
| UCTD | 9 (2) | 9 (1.4) | (2) | — |
| Overlap | — | 14 (2.2) | — | 29 (9.0) |
| Other | — | 3 (0.5) | (15) | 23 (7.2) |
| Unknown | — | 7 (1.0) | — | — |
| Total | 429 (100) | 641 (100) | 129 (100) | 321 (100) |

*Abbreviations:* DM, dermatomyositis; MCTD, mixed connective tissue disease; PAH, pulmonary arterial hypertension; PM, polymyositis; pSS, primary Sjogren's syndrome; RA, rheumatoid arthritis; SLE, systemic lupus erythematosus; SSc, systemic sclerosis; UCTD, undifferentiated connective tissue disease.
[a] Only 24 patients had PAH confirmed by right heart catheterization.
[b] Of the 399 patients with SSc, 251 (63%) had limited SSc, 77 (19%) had diffuse SSc, 71 (18%) were unspecified.

they defined a patient as having PH or PAH with an RVSP of greater than 30 mm Hg. Current clinical guidelines for PH recommend further workup for PH in a patient with unexplained dyspnea when the RVSP is greater than 40 mm Hg.[12]

### Systemic Sclerosis

Current estimates report that the prevalence of RHC-confirmed PAH in SSc is 7.85% to 13% of patients.[13–15] The DETECT study is a large cross-sectional study of SSc to develop a detection algorithm for PAH. The authors included 466 patients who had SSc for longer than 3 years and a diffusing capacity of carbon monoxide (DLCO) of less than 60% who then underwent a panel of screening tests, echocardiography, and RHC. Of this group, 19% of patients were found to have RHC-confirmed PAH.[16]

The incidence of PAH was estimated in the ItinerAIR-Sclerodermie Study, a prospective cohort study of SSc patients without significant left heart disease or ILD. Patients were routinely screened with echocardiogram, and those with a velocity of tricuspid regurgitation of greater than 3.0 m/s or a velocity of tricuspid regurgitation of 2.8 to 3.0 m/s with unexplained dyspnea were considered to screen positively and underwent RHC. Of 384 patients followed over a median of 41 months, 8 patients were found to have PAH, which is an incidence of 0.61 cases per 100 patient-years.[17]

### Systemic Lupus Erythematosus, Mixed Connective Tissue Diseases, and Other Connective Tissue Diseases

In a large registry of SLE patients in China, the prevalence of PAH by echocardiogram (criteria for defining PAH was not reported) was 3.8%.[18] Another study with a cohort of patients from Spain screened SLE patients with serial echocardiograms. Patients who had 2 echocardiograms with a PASP of 40 mm Hg or greater underwent RHC. Of the 245 patients included, 12 cases of PH were diagnosed, corresponding to a prevalence of 5%.[19]

There are few data on the prevalence of PH in MCTD. A recent study screened a cohort of 147 Norwegian MCTD patients with echocardiograms and performed RHC if the RVSP was greater than 40 mm Hg. They found that only 5 patients (3.4%) developed PH over a median follow-up of 5.6 years, and that only 2 of 5 had PAH, whereas the other 3 had PH with ILD.[20]

The published studies on the frequency of PAH in other CTDs report a relatively high prevalence, but are all based on echocardiographic measures without confirmation by RHC. Because these other CTDs only account for a small portion of CTD-PAH patients, it is generally thought that PAH is associated only rarely with these diagnoses.

The prevalence of PH in RA has been estimated at 20% to 26.7% based on 3 cohort studies of RA patients who underwent screening echocardiograms. In all 3 studies, PH was defined as a PASP of greater than 30 mm Hg and was considered PAH if there was no evidence for underlying ILD or left heart disease. Notably, in all 3 studies, the majority of patients with PH had a PASP between 30 and 40 mm Hg, and out of the 50 patients combined from all 3 studies, only 2 patients had a PASP of greater than 50 mm Hg.[21–23]

Aside from 1 small study, there are few data on the prevalence of dermatomyositis/PM–associated PH. In that study, a retrospective cohort of 30 Jordanian patients with dermatomyositis/PM was analyzed. Nineteen patients underwent echocardiogram and 3 were found to have PH based on an RVSP of greater than 40 mm Hg.[24]

The prevalence of PH in pSS has also been reported to be greater than 20%. In 1 study, 24 of 107 pSS patients were found to have PH as defined by a PASP of greater than 35 mm Hg, although for most patients, PH was mild.[25] Only 3 patients had a PASP of greater than 50 mm Hg and one of these patients had ILD. Another, similar study examined 47 patients with pSS with screening echocardiography and PH was defined as a PASP of greater than 30 mm Hg. In this cohort, 11 of the 47 patients (23.4%) screened positively, although 6 of the 11 had a PASP between 30 and 35 mm Hg.[26]

## PATHOLOGY AND PATHOPHYSIOLOGY

As stated, PAH is a disease characterized by vasoconstriction and remodeling of the small to medium sized pulmonary arterioles. Abnormalities in all layers of the vasculature have been noted: proliferation of endothelial cells and intimal thickening, medial hypertrophy, and thickening of the adventitia. Although all forms of PAH exhibit these pathologic findings, a recent study describes a unique pattern in CTD-PAH with areas of marked interstitial inflammation and fibrotic changes.[3]

Preclinical studies support the concept that PAH may be triggered by immune dysregulation. For example, athymic rats, which lack T cells, can develop severe PH under normoxic conditions when treated with the vascular endothelial growth factor receptor-2 antagonist, SU5416.[27] Moreover, the development of PH in this model can be attenuated by immune reconstitution with regulatory T cells.[28]

Autoantibodies, specifically anti-endothelial cell antibodies (AECAs), have also been implicated in the pathogenesis of PAH. AECAs are a group of autoantibodies that target endothelial cells and may lead to endothelial injury. Ex vivo assays of anti-endothelial cell immunoglobulin (Ig)G or IgM antibodies show that they engage endothelial cells, activate complement pathways and platelet binding,[29] and induce endothelial cell apoptosis.[30–34] Several studies have established an association between serum AECAs and the severity of disease activity in SLE and SSc.[35–38] For example, patients with SSc and SLE with IgG-specific AECAs had a higher incidence of PAH compared with patients with no detectable antibodies. Based on the positive correlation between the degree of PAH and the staining intensity of the assay, it has been hypothesized that AECAs may trigger PAH in some patients. In another study, 76 patients with SSc and 50 matched healthy controls were examined and those with AECAs had a significantly higher incidence of digital infarcts, gangrene, and PAH than those without these antibodies.[35] Last, a recent study from China measured the presence of pulmonary arterial AECAs in the serum of 19 CTD-PAH patients compared with 22 CTD patients without PAH, and normal controls. They found that 63% of the CTD-PAH patients had elevated levels of AECAs compared with 40% of the patients with CTDs but no PAH, and only 5% of the healthy controls. Moreover, the level of AECAs was significantly higher in the CTD-PAH patients compared with the CTD patients without PAH.[39]

Another inflammatory mediator that has been implicated in the pathogenesis of CTD-PAH is leukotriene $B_4$ ($LTB_4$). A recent study demonstrated that patients with CTD-PAH had elevated serum levels of $LTB_4$ compared with healthy controls and patients with idiopathic PAH (IPAH), and that the plexiform lesions of patients with CTD-PAH had increased numbers of $LTB_4$ secreting macrophages.[40] This study went on to show that $LTB_4$ promoted endothelial cell apoptosis and pulmonary artery smooth muscle cell proliferation, and that inhibition of $LTB_4$ in a rat model of severe PH attenuated the disease and reversed pulmonary vascular remodeling.

Thrombosis is a common histologic finding in the pulmonary vasculature of patients with CTD-PAH.[3] However, it is unclear whether this is secondary to the endothelial dysfunction and the underlying disease, or if this is a primary pathogenic process that contributes to pulmonary vascular remodeling.

In addition to the mediators described that may contribute to the pathogenesis of CTD-PAH, some mediators have been implicated in the pathogenesis of SSc-PAH specifically. A recent proteome-wide analysis of plasmacytoid dendritic cells, the cells responsible for the production of type I interferon, identified CXCL4, a potent anti-angiogenic chemokine, as a predominant protein secreted by these cells in SSc patients. High levels of CXCL4 expression in the serum correlated strongly with the development of PAH. Interestingly, in vitro studies demonstrated that CXCL4 induced human umbilical vein endothelial cells to secrete endothelin-1, a potent vasoconstrictor known to contribute to the pathophysiology of PAH.[41]

One recent study suggests that dysregulation of bone morphogenetic protein receptor 2 (BMPR2) may contribute to SSc-PAH pathogenesis. BMPR2 is a receptor in the transforming growth factor-β family of receptors and mutations in this gene cause a hereditary form of PAH. It is an autosomal-dominant mutation, but has only a 20% penetrance. This study examined microvascular endothelial cells from patients with SSc and found that the cells had significantly decreased expression levels of BMPR2 and were more sensitive to apoptotic signals. Moreover, they found that the SSc endothelial cells had extensive CpG sites of methylation in the BMPR2 promoter region, likely leading to repression of BMPR2 expression.[42]

Anti-U1 ribonucleoprotein (RNP) antibodies are present in up to 18% and 12% of patients with SSc and SLE, respectively, and high titers characterize patients with MCTD.[43,44] These antibodies are thought to contribute to PAH pathogenesis by inducing endothelial cell activation and damage. One study demonstrated that the supernatant from monocytes stimulated with anti–U1-RNP antibodies increased interleukin (IL)-1α and IL-6 production from human pulmonary artery endothelial cells, suggesting that anti–U1-RNP stimulates the production of cytokines that activate human pulmonary artery endothelial cells.[45]

## RISK FACTORS AND PREDICTORS FOR THE DEVELOPMENT OF PULMONARY ARTERIAL HYPERTENSION
### Systemic Sclerosis

The risk of developing SSc-PAH is greater in older patients and patients who have had a longer duration of disease.[14] Other clinical features that have been associated with a risk for developing PAH include severe Raynaud phenomenon and the presence of digital ulcers.[46] An isolated decreased DLCO has been found to be a strong risk factor and predictor of PAH in SSc.[46–48] Allanore and colleagues[48] reported that by using a cutoff of DLCO/VA (alveolar volume) of less than 60% predicted had a hazard ratio of 36.66 for the development of SSc-PAH. Elevated N-terminal brain natriuretic peptide (NT-proBNP) levels have also been shown in multiple studies to be a predictor for the development of SSc-PAH. In a prospective study of SSc patients, NT-proBNP levels that were greater than 97th percentile of normal values based on age and sex were associated with a hazard ratio of 9.97 for the development of PAH.[48]

The rate of increase in RVSP on echocardiogram has also been shown to be a predictor for the development of PAH in SSc patients. An RVSP increase of 1 to 1.99 mm Hg per year corresponded with a hazard ratio of 1.9, an increase of 2 to 2.99 mm Hg per year corresponded with a hazard ratio of 5.09, and a rate of increase of greater than 3 mm Hg per year yielded a hazard ratio of 6.15 for the development of PAH over a mean follow-up time of 7.7 years.[49]

Borderline elevations in mPAP have been shown to be a risk factor for the eventual development of PAH. In a study of 228 SSc patients who had been screened previously for PAH with an RHC, 142 patients had a normal mPAP of less than 20 mm Hg, and 86 patients had a borderline mPAP of 21 to 24 mm Hg. For patients who met prespecified criteria, 38 patients with previously normal mPAP and 38 patients with previously borderline mPAP underwent repeat RHC. Of the 38 patients with a borderline mPAP, 16 were diagnosed with PAH on the follow-up RHC compared with only 7 patients with a previously normal RHC.[50] This corresponded with a hazard ratio of 3.7 for developing PAH if one had a borderline mPAP. This study also found that the risk of developing PAH was predicted by having an elevated transpulmonary gradient (the difference between the mPAP and pulmonary artery wedge pressure) of greater than 11 mm Hg, with a hazard ratio of 7.9. Another study demonstrated that CTD patients with borderline elevations in mPAP had a decreased survival compared with non-CTD patients.[51]

Specific autoantibody profiles have been associated with an increased risk for the development of SSc-PAH. Specifically, the absence of anti-scl 70 antibody portends a greater risk, whereas the presence of anti-centromere, anti-U1RNP, nucleolar ANA, and anti-phospholipid antibodies denote a higher risk profile.[52] Some novel antibodies have also been associated with an increased risk of PAH, including AECA and anti-4-sulfated N-acetyllactosamine antibodies.

Other inflammatory mediators have been associated with SSc-PAH. One study examined the cytokine profiles of SSc patients and correlated them with clinical features. The authors found that SSc patients with PH tended to have higher levels of IL-6 and IL-13 compared with SSc patients without PH. The calculated odds ratio for PH was 1.31 and 1.42 for IL-6 and IL-13, respectively.[53] Another recent study examined the serum concentrations of soluble CD90, a soluble adhesion molecule secreted from activated endothelial cells that is involved in leukocyte recruitment, in patients with SSc. They found that patients with PAH had significantly elevated soluble CD90 compared with SSc patients without PAH.[54]

## Systemic Lupus Erythematosus

A retrospective study of 93 French SLE patients found that 9 patients likely had PAH based on a PASP of 35 mm Hg or greater on echocardiogram. Clinical features associated with an increased risk for the development of SLE-PAH included black race, longer disease duration, pericarditis, and a history of peripheral nervous system involvement.[55] Another relatively large cohort study of 288 SLE patients from the UK found 12 patients with PH based on an echocardiogram with an RVSP of greater than 30 mm Hg. Antiphospholipid antibody syndrome had a borderline correlation with the development of PH,[56] with a positive lupus anticoagulant in 55% of the SLE-PH patients, compared with only 16% of the patients without PH.[56] PH patients were also more likely to be anti-La positive (50%) compared with non-PH patients (21%).[56] Fois and colleagues[55] found that SLE patients with PH defined by PASP on echocardiogram of 35 mm Hg or greater tended to be anti-Sm antibody and anti-cardiolipin antibody positive.

## Other Connective Tissue Diseases

One study found that the development of PH in pSS was strongly correlated with the presence of lung disease, interstitial nephritis, cryoglobulinemia, and hypocomplementemia.[25] A second study reported increased risk of PH with pSS in patients who were younger and with a shorter disease duration.[26]

## SCREENING FOR PULMONARY ARTERIAL HYPERTENSION

Current guidelines recommend that patients with SSc spectrum disorders, specifically, SSc, MCTD, and other CTDs with a predominance of SSc features, undergo annual screening for PAH with echocardiograms.[1] Routine screening for PAH in other

CTDs is not recommended currently.[1] However, as described, RVSP or PASP measures on echocardiogram do not always correlate well with RHC measures, so a number of studies have examined the utility of additional factors that may be used for screening either alone or in combination with echocardiography. As stated, both DLCO and NT-proBNP have been found to be strong predictors for SSc-PAH and have been included in several screening algorithms.

A recent systematic review evaluated the performance of different screening algorithms for SSc-PAH.[57] The authors included only studies of SSc patients without previously diagnosed PAH and PAH confirmed by RHC. Nine studies with a total intent-to-screen population of 3504 patients were included. In studies of prevalent disease, the positive predictive value of screening ranged from 20.4% to 87.0%, and the positive predictive value of screening for incident disease ranged from 20.0% to 30.7%.

The shortcomings of current screening algorithms highlighted by this study may be at least partially obviated by the recently published DETECT study.[16] This study examined 466 patients with SSc of at least 3 years duration and a DLCO of less than 60% predicted. All of these patients underwent a broad assessment including serum testing, electrocardiogram, echocardiogram, and RHC. From these data, a 2-step algorithm was developed to determine which patients should undergo a screening echocardiogram and which patients should proceed to RHC (**Fig. 1**). Step 1 includes 6 simple assessments that are used to calculate a score that determines whether a patient goes on to echocardiography. In step 2, the step 1 score and 2

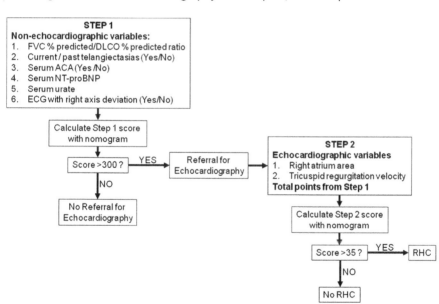

**Fig. 1.** DETECT algorithm for screening for systemic sclerosis pulmonary arterial hypertension (SSc-PAH). SSc patients are screened with the 6 assessments in step 1. A nomogram is used to calculate the score of step 1 and if the score is greater than 300, the patient is referred for echocardiogram. In step 2, the step 1 score and 2 echocardiographic measures are used to calculate a score with the step 2 nomogram. If the score is greater than 35, the patient is referred for RHC. ACA, anticentromere antibody; DLCO, diffusion capacity of carbon monoxide; ECG, electrocardiogram; FVC, forced vital capacity; NT-proBNP, N terminal brain natriuretic peptide; RHC, right heart catheterization. (*Adapted from* Coghlan JG, Denton CP, Grunig E, et al. Evidence-based detection of pulmonary arterial hypertension in systemic sclerosis: the DETECT study. Ann Rheum Dis 2014;73:1340–49.)

echocardiographic parameters are used to determine which patients should undergo RHC. The sensitivity of detecting PAH with this algorithm was 96%. This algorithm has yet to be validated in a prospective cohort.

## CLINICAL PRESENTATION AND EVALUATION

The presentation of CTD-PAH is similar to that of other forms of PAH. The most commonly reported symptoms are dyspnea on exertion and decreased exercise tolerance. Other common symptoms include fatigue and weakness. Patients may also report chest pain, palpitations, or lightheadedness with activity. Syncopal episodes are a sign of severe disease. Patients with CTD-PAH usually carry a CTD diagnosis before presentation with PAH, although, on occasion, PAH can be the presenting sign of a CTD.[58,59]

Most patients with CTDs who present for evaluation for PAH will already have had a screening echocardiogram. For each of these patients, a full diagnostic workup for PH should be completed. Although the CTD will be the mostly likely cause of PH in these patients, they may have other risk factors and comorbid conditions that might contribute.

Initial evaluation should include a full history and physical examination. Specific attention should be made for any family history of PH, personal or family history of thromboembolic disease, risk factors for human immunodeficiency virus or liver disease, and any history of anorexigen or stimulant use. Physical examination should assess for signs of right heart failure, such as elevated jugular venous pulsation and lower extremity edema. On cardiac examination, patients often have a prominent second heart sound and may also have a tricuspid regurgitant murmur, an S4, and/or a laterally displaced point of maximal impulse. Lung examination in patients without concomitant ILD is usually normal.

Most CTD patients on presentation will already have had a full set of pulmonary function tests with DLCO and autoimmune serologies. Additional diagnostic testing should include a human immunodeficiency virus and liver function tests, VQ scan to evaluate for chronic thromboembolic disease, overnight oximetry and/or polysomnography to assess for sleep apnea, and a 6-minute walk test and/or cardiopulmonary exercise test to assess functional capacity.[1,12] Supplemental testing, including echocardiography with bubble study to assess for shunt, CT angiography, pulmonary angiogram, and hypercoaguable panel for chronic thromboembolic disease, may be indicated. Last, all patients should undergo RHC to confirm the diagnosis. RHC should include measurements of right atrial pressure, right ventricular pressure, PAP, pulmonary artery wedge pressure, and cardiac output.[12] Previous guidelines had recommended an acute vasodilator challenge in all patients with a new diagnosis of PAH. For this test, patients are given a vasodilator such as inhaled nitric oxide or intravenous adenosine or epoprostenol. A positive vasodilator response is defined as a decrease in the mPAP by greater than 10 mm Hg, to a mPAP of less than 40 mm Hg, with a stable or improved cardiac output. A positive response identifies patients with a better prognosis and those who are likely to respond to therapy with oral calcium channel blockers.[12] However, studies have shown that a positive vasodilator response is exceedingly rare in CTD-PAH, such that most recent consensus statements recommend performing this test only for "scientific purposes."[1]

## MANAGEMENT OF CONNECTIVE TISSUE DISEASE–ASSOCIATED PULMONARY ARTERIAL HYPERTENSION
### Pulmonary Vasodilators

Once a diagnosis of PAH is confirmed by RHC, treatment with pulmonary vasodilators should be initiated. Currently, there are 4 classes of pulmonary vasodilators that target

3 pathways. The phosphodiesterase-5 inhibitors and soluble guanylate cyclase stimulators are oral medications that target the nitric oxide pathway and act to increase the concentration of nitric oxide and hence promote vasodilation in the pulmonary vasculature. The endothelin receptor antagonists are oral therapies that block the binding of endothelin-1 to its receptor to prevent endothelin-mediated vasoconstriction. Last, the prostacyclin analogs act on the prostacyclin pathway to stimulate cyclic adenosine monophosphate, which promotes vasodilation. Prostacyclin analogs are available as continuous intravenous (IV) or subcutaneous infusions, inhaled, or oral forms (**Box 2**). Patients with CTD-PAH were included in all of the phase 3, randomized, controlled trials for PAH-specific therapies, so these diagnoses are US Food and Drug Administration–approved indications for these medications. A recent meta-analysis of 9 clinical trials of CTD-PAH patients analyzed the improvement in 6-minute walk distance with pulmonary vasodilators. The authors found that the improvement in 6-minute walk distance with phosphodiesterase-5 inhibitors was 37 to 47 m, with ERAs was 14.1 to 21.7 m, and with prostacyclins was 21 to 108 m. With this, they concluded that these 3 classes of medications were effective in CTD-PAH, but perhaps ERAs were less effective.[60]

Current treatment guidelines are generalized for all group 1 PAH with no distinct recommendations for CTD-PAH.[7,61] The primary basis for initial therapy is World Health Organization (WHO) functional class (FC; analogous to New York Heart Association Functional Class [NYHA FC]). In general, patients with WHO FC 2 symptoms, that

---

**Box 2**
**US Food and Drug Administration–approved therapies for PAH: Current PAH-specific therapies target 3 pathways**

*Nitric oxide pathway*

Phosphodiesterase-5 inhibitors (PDE-5i)

   Sildenafil

   Tadalafil

Soluble guanylate cyclase stimulators

   Riociguat

*Endothelin pathway*

Endothelin receptor antagonists (ERA)

   Bosentan

   Ambrisentan

   Macitentan

*Prostacyclin pathway*

Prostacyclin analogs

   Epoprostenol IV

   Treprostinil IV, SC, INH, PO

   Iloprost INH

*Abbreviations:* INH, inhaled; IV, intravenous; PAH, pulmonary arterial hypertension; PO, oral; SC, subcutaneous.
*Data from* Galie N, Corris PA, Frost A, et al. Updated treatment algorithm of pulmonary arterial hypertension. J Am Coll Cardiol 2013;62:D60–72.

is, symptoms with normal physical activity, may be initiated with oral therapy, whereas patients with WHO FC 4 status, that is, symptoms at rest or syncope, should be started on continuous infusion prostacyclin therapy. Patients with WHO FC 3 symptoms, that is, symptoms with less than ordinary activity, may be started on either oral therapy or parenteral therapy. The recent CHEST guidelines recommend the use of parenteral therapy for WHO FC 3 patients with rapid progression of disease or markers of poor clinical prognosis.[61] Because of a lack of head-to-head trials for most therapies, the World Symposium on PH guidelines give few recommendations for choosing one agent over another, whereas the CHEST guidelines offer narrow suggestions based on the available data from controlled studies.[7,61] As a result, decisions around initial therapy are often driven by local expertise and practice patterns, patient preference, and insurance considerations. Regardless of initial therapy, the current guidelines recommend that, if patients have an inadequate response to therapy, combination therapy should be initiated. Given the poor prognosis of patients with CTD-PAH, particularly SSc-PAH, aggressive initiation and escalation of therapy should be considered.

### Supportive Therapy

In addition to pulmonary vasodilators, some supportive therapies are recommended. Patients should receive routine vaccinations. Patients who are hypoxic with an oxygen saturation of less than 88% on room air at rest, with activity, or with sleep, should be given supplemental oxygen. Diuretics should be used to manage symptoms of volume overload from right heart failure. Digoxin may be helpful for increasing right ventricular contractility. Last, women of childbearing age should be counseled against pregnancy, because this is associated with a mortality rate of 15% to 30%.[7]

As stated, there is evidence for pulmonary vascular thrombosis in the pathology of patients with PAH. Anticoagulation in IPAH has been shown in a number of studies to improve survival,[62] but its role in other forms of PAH including CTD-PAH remains unclear. Given the association of CTDs, especially SLE, with antiphospholipid antibodies and the risk of thrombosis, there is some clinical rationale for the use of anticoagulation in CTD-PAH. However, current guidelines rate anticoagulation in associated PAH as a IIb recommendation.[7] A retrospective study of the COMPERA registry examined the survival of group 1 PAH patients with or without anticoagulation. There was no improvement in survival in non-IPAH patients with anticoagulation. The authors analyzed the subgroup of 208 patients with SSc-PAH, 50% of whom were on anticoagulation. The 3-year survival for patients on anticoagulation was 62.7% compared with 73.7% for the group not on anticoagulation ($P = .28$).[62] Conversely, a recent study of 117 CTD-PAH patients, 95% of whom had SSc, treated with pulmonary vasodilators, demonstrated a significant survival benefit in patients treated with warfarin. This study reported a 5-fold reduction in mortality over a mean of 2.6 years with the use of anticoagulation.[63]

### Immunosuppression

Overall, there are currently no specific guidelines for the use of immunosuppressants for CTD-PAH. A number of case series have reported the use of aggressive immunosuppression for the treatment of CTD-PAH. Sanchez and colleagues[64] studied 28 patients with CTD-PAH and treated them with IV cyclophosphamide monotherapy with or without high-dose glucocorticoids alone for at least 3 months, or in combination with PAH-specific therapies. Eight (5 SLE-PAH and 3 MCTD-PAH) of 28 patients responded to therapy with immunosuppression as defined by improvement in hemodynamics and NYHA FC to either class 1 or 2 after at least 1 year. None of the

SSc-PAH patients responded to immunotherapy. Response to immunosuppression also correlated with improved survival. A similar Japanese study treated a group of 13 patients with CTD-PAH with IV cyclophosphamide and glucocorticoids for 12 to 18 months in addition to pulmonary vasodilators.[65] Compared with historical controls, the immunosuppression group had a significant decrease in mPAP and had improved survival. Moreover, 6 of the 13 patients had near normalization of their mPAP that was maintained for at least 12 months. Like the study from Sanchez and colleagues, the 1 patient with SSc-PAH did not respond to immunosuppression. Another study of immunosuppression in CTD-PAH focused on just SLE-PAH and MCTD-PAH patients.[66] Sixteen patients were treated with IV cyclophosphamide for 6 months and glucocorticoids for at least 4 weeks, whereas 8 patients were treated with immunosuppression along with PAH-specific therapies. Of the patients treated with immunosuppression alone, 8 patients (50%) were deemed to be responders to therapy as defined by improvements in hemodynamics defined as an mPAP of less than 40 mm Hg and/or normal cardiac index, and an NYHA FC of 1 or 2.

In all 3 of these studies, patients who responded to immunosuppressive therapy tended to have less severe disease at baseline. In the studies by Sanchez and colleagues[64] and Jais and colleagues,[66] responders had a better WHO FC, higher cardiac index, and/or lower pulmonary vascular resistance index at presentation. In the study from Japan, aside from 1 patient who presented with a mPAP in the 60s, responders tended to have lower mPAPs at presentation. This pattern suggests that patients may be more likely to respond to immunosuppressive therapy at an earlier phase of the disease, potentially because those with longstanding PAH have developed irreversible pathologic changes of their pulmonary vessels.[67] However, it should be noted that at least in the study by Sanchez and colleagues there were no differences in the mean time between diagnosis of CTDs and PAH or mean delay between PAH diagnosis and initiation of immunosuppressive therapy in responders compared with nonresponders.

There is some evidence that shorter courses of high-dose immunosuppression may be effective for the treatment of CTD-PAH. A case series of 4 patients with SLE-PAH and 1 patient with PM-PAH reported that treatment with high dose prednisolone or methylprednisolone for 2 to 4 weeks led to improvement in WHO FC in all patients within 4 weeks. Moreover, the reduction in steroid dose in 2 patients was associated with worsening FC and required escalation of pulmonary vasodilator therapy.[68]

There are few data on the use of immunosuppressants other than cyclophosphamide and glucocorticoids for CTD-PAH. Two animal studies have suggested that mycophenolate mofetil (MMF) may be beneficial for PAH. Rats with PH induced with monocrotaline were treated with MMF at either 20 or 40 mg/kg per day or a vehicle control. The rats treated with MMF had a significant reduction in RVSP, right ventricular hypertrophy, and reduced medial wall thickness of the pulmonary arterioles. This was also associated with decreases in the infiltration of macrophages, proliferating cell nuclear antigen–positive cells, and expression of P-selectin and IL-6.[69] A second study also demonstrated that MMF was associated with a decrease in RVSP, decrease in arteriole wall thickness, and infiltration of inflammatory cells. This study went on to show that both the proliferation and viability of pulmonary artery smooth muscle cells were inhibited by MMF.[70] One report of 2 patients with SLE-PAH reported that treatment with dexamethasone and methotrexate followed by maintenance therapy with cyclosporine and steroids led to a reduction in RVSP, improvement in right ventricular function, and improvement in functional status.[71] Another agent that has been reported to successfully treat SSc, MCTD, and SLE-PAH is rituximab.[72–74] Studies have shown that it can be an effective therapy for SSc-ILD and skin fibrosis.[75,76] Based on these reports and preclinical data, a National Institutes of Health–sponsored, placebo-controlled clinical trial of rituximab for the treatment of SSc-PAH is currently underway (ClinicalTrials.gov identifier: NCT01086540).

## PROGNOSIS
### Systemic Sclerosis

PAH accounts for 14% of deaths in SSc and is the second leading cause of mortality in these patients after ILD.[77,78] In an early cohort study of SSc-PAH during which pulmonary vasodilators were not widely available, the 1-, 2-, and 3-year survival rates were 81%, 63%, and 56%, respectively.[13] Unfortunately, although there have been appreciable reductions in mortality in all-comers with PAH in the modern era of PAH therapy, there has been little improvement in survival in SSc-PAH. From the REVEAL registry, 3-year survival in patients with SSc-PAH was 61.4%, whereas the survival of patients with newly diagnosed SSc-PAH was poor at only 51%. This was significantly worse compared with the non-SSc CTD-PAH cohort in whom 3-year survival was 80.9% overall and 76.4% in newly diagnosed patients.[79] The UK CTD-PAH and French cohorts had similar findings in SSc-PAH with 3-year survivals of 47% and 56%, respectively.[6,80] In the Australian Scleroderma Cohort Study, the median survival for SSc-PAH was only 5 years.[8] A recent meta-analysis of 22 studies of SSc-PAH found that the pooled 1-, 2-, and 3-year survivals were 81%, 64%, and 52%, respectively, and that the meta-regression did not reveal a significant change in survival over time.[81] Interestingly, a study from the Pulmonary Hypertension Assessment and Recognition of Outcomes in Scleroderma (PHAROS) registry found that in 131 patients with incident PAH, 1-, 2-, and 3-year survival rates were better at 93%, 88%, and 75%, respectively.[82] Because PHAROS is a registry of SSc patients at high risk for PAH who are being screened for PAH, improvement in survival may be attributed to earlier detection of disease. This is supported by the finding that patients had a better FC at diagnosis: 56% of patients were WHO FC 1 or 2 compared with only 23% in the REVEAL registry. However, improved survival related to lead time bias cannot be excluded.

### Systemic Lupus Erythematosus

Aside from 1 study that reported a 3-year survival rate of SLE-PH patients of only 44.9%,[83] current data suggest that SLE-PAH patients experience better survival than those with SSc-PAH. In the UK CTD-PAH cohort, 3-year survival of SLE-PAH was 75%,[6] whereas in a Chinese cohort of CTD-PAH, the SLE-PAH patients had a 3-year survival of 88%.[9] Similar results were obtained with analysis of the REVEAL registry, 1-year survival was 94% and 2-year survival was 85%.[5]

### Mixed Connective Tissue Disease and Other Connective Tissue Diseases

Data from the REVEAL registry suggests that survival in MCTD-PAH is similar to that of SSc-PAH with a 1-year survival of 88% and 2-year survival of 72%.[5] This study also reported a 1-year survival of 96% for RA-PAH.[5] There are few data on the survival rate of pSS patients with PAH. One case series reported a 1-year survival of only 73% and a 3-year survival of 66%.[84]

## SUMMARY

PAH is a serious complication of CTDs and accounts for a substantial portion of the associated morbidity and mortality. In recent years, much work has been done to characterize the phenotype of CTD-PAH, not only how it differs from IPAH, but also how different subtypes of CTD-PAH differ from each other. Numerous epidemiologic studies, including several large international registries, have helped to clarify the burden of disease. Unfortunately, although the advent of specific therapies for PAH has led to significant improvements in survival in IPAH patients, some subsets of CTD-PAH, particularly SSc-PAH, have not had any appreciable improvement in survival with therapy. Novel screening algorithms for PAH in SSc patients may allow potentially earlier detection and improved survival in this subgroup. In addition, further research on pathogenetic mechanisms of CTD-PAH will hopefully identify novel therapeutic targets for these patients.

## REFERENCES

1. Hoeper MM, Bogaard HJ, Condliffe R, et al. Definitions and diagnosis of pulmonary hypertension. J Am Coll Cardiol 2013;62:D42–50.
2. Simonneau G, Gatzoulis MA, Adatia I, et al. Updated clinical classification of pulmonary hypertension. J Am Coll Cardiol 2013;62:D34–41.
3. Stacher E, Graham BB, Hunt JM, et al. Modern age pathology of pulmonary arterial hypertension. Am J Respir Crit Care Med 2012;186:261–72.
4. D'Alonzo GE, Barst RJ, Ayres SM, et al. Survival in patients with primary pulmonary hypertension. Results from a national prospective registry. Ann Intern Med 1991;115:343–9.
5. Chung L, Liu J, Parsons L, et al. Characterization of connective tissue disease-associated pulmonary arterial hypertension from REVEAL: identifying systemic sclerosis as a unique phenotype. Chest 2010;138:1383–94.
6. Condliffe R, Kiely DG, Peacock AJ, et al. Connective tissue disease-associated pulmonary arterial hypertension in the modern treatment era. Am J Respir Crit Care Med 2009;179:151–7.
7. Galie N, Corris PA, Frost A, et al. Updated treatment algorithm of pulmonary arterial hypertension. J Am Coll Cardiol 2013;62:D60–72.
8. Ngian GS, Stevens W, Prior D, et al. Predictors of mortality in connective tissue disease-associated pulmonary arterial hypertension: a cohort study. Arthritis Res Ther 2012;14:R213.
9. Hao YJ, Jiang X, Zhou W, et al. Connective tissue disease-associated pulmonary arterial hypertension in Chinese patients. Eur Respir J 2014;44:963–72.
10. Jeon CH, Chai JY, Seo YI, et al. Pulmonary hypertension associated with rheumatic diseases: baseline characteristics from the Korean registry. Int J Rheum Dis 2012;15:e80–9.
11. Finkelhor RS, Lewis SA, Pillai D. Limitations and strengths of Doppler/echo pulmonary artery systolic pressure-right heart catheterization correlations: a systematic literature review. Echocardiography 2014;32:10–8.
12. McLaughlin VV, Archer SL, Badesch DB, et al. ACCF/AHA 2009 expert consensus document on pulmonary hypertension: a report of the American College of Cardiology Foundation Task Force on Expert Consensus Documents and the American Heart Association: developed in collaboration with the American College of Chest Physicians, American Thoracic Society, Inc., and the Pulmonary Hypertension Association. Circulation 2009;119:2250–94.
13. Mukerjee D, St George D, Coleiro B, et al. Prevalence and outcome in systemic sclerosis associated pulmonary arterial hypertension: application of a registry approach. Ann Rheum Dis 2003;62:1088–93.

14. Hachulla E, Gressin V, Guillevin L, et al. Early detection of pulmonary arterial hypertension in systemic sclerosis: a French nationwide prospective multicenter study. Arthritis Rheum 2005;52:3792–800.

15. Phung S, Strange G, Chung LP, et al. Prevalence of pulmonary arterial hypertension in an Australian scleroderma population: screening allows for earlier diagnosis. Intern Med J 2009;39:682–91.

16. Coghlan JG, Denton CP, Grunig E, et al. Evidence-based detection of pulmonary arterial hypertension in systemic sclerosis: the DETECT study. Ann Rheum Dis 2014;73:1340–9.

17. Hachulla E, de Groote P, Gressin V, et al. The three-year incidence of pulmonary arterial hypertension associated with systemic sclerosis in a multicenter nationwide longitudinal study in France. Arthritis Rheum 2009;60:1831–9.

18. Li M, Zhang W, Leng X, et al. Chinese SLE Treatment and Research group (CSTAR) registry: I. major clinical characteristics of Chinese patients with systemic lupus erythematosus. Lupus 2013;22:1192–9.

19. Ruiz-Irastorza G, Garmendia M, Villar I, et al. Pulmonary hypertension in systemic lupus erythematosus: prevalence, predictors and diagnostic strategy. Autoimmun Rev 2013;12:410–5.

20. Gunnarsson R, Andreassen AK, Molberg O, et al. Prevalence of pulmonary hypertension in an unselected, mixed connective tissue disease cohort: results of a nationwide, Norwegian cross-sectional multicentre study and review of current literature. Rheumatology 2013;52:1208–13.

21. Dawson JK, Goodson NG, Graham DR, et al. Raised pulmonary artery pressures measured with Doppler echocardiography in rheumatoid arthritis patients. Rheumatology 2000;39:1320–5.

22. Keser G, Capar I, Aksu K, et al. Pulmonary hypertension in rheumatoid arthritis. Scand J Rheumatol 2004;33:244–5.

23. Udayakumar N, Venkatesan S, Rajendiran C. Pulmonary hypertension in rheumatoid arthritis–relation with the duration of the disease. Int J Cardiol 2008;127:410–2.

24. Mustafa KN, Dahbour SS. Clinical characteristics and outcomes of patients with idiopathic inflammatory myopathies from Jordan 1996-2009. Clin Rheumatol 2010;29:1381–5.

25. Vassiliou VA, Moyssakis I, Boki KA, et al. Is the heart affected in primary Sjogren's syndrome? An echocardiographic study. Clin Exp Rheumatol 2008;26:109–12.

26. Kobak S, Kalkan S, Kirilmaz B, et al. Pulmonary arterial hypertension in patients with primary Sjogren's syndrome. Autoimmune Dis 2014;2014:710401.

27. Taraseviciene-Stewart L, Nicolls MR, Kraskauskas D, et al. Absence of T cells confers increased pulmonary arterial hypertension and vascular remodeling. Am J Respir Crit Care Med 2007;175:1280–9.

28. Tamosiuniene R, Tian W, Dhillon G, et al. Regulatory T cells limit vascular endothelial injury and prevent pulmonary hypertension. Circ Res 2011;109:867–79.

29. Cines DB, Lyss AP, Reeber M, et al. Presence of complement-fixing anti-endothelial cell antibodies in systemic lupus erythematosus. J Clin Invest 1984;73:611–25.

30. Dieude M, Senecal JL, Raymond Y. Induction of endothelial cell apoptosis by heat-shock protein 60-reactive antibodies from anti-endothelial cell autoantibody-positive systemic lupus erythematosus patients. Arthritis Rheum 2004;50:3221–31.

31. Worda M, Sgonc R, Dietrich H, et al. In vivo analysis of the apoptosis-inducing effect of anti-endothelial cell antibodies in systemic sclerosis by the chorionallantoic membrane assay. Arthritis Rheum 2003;48:2605–14.

32. Bordron A, Dueymes M, Levy Y, et al. The binding of some human antiendothelial cell antibodies induces endothelial cell apoptosis. J Clin Invest 1998;101: 2029–35.

33. Kaneko K, Savage CO, Pottinger BE, et al. Antiendothelial cell antibodies can be cytotoxic to endothelial cells without cytokine pre-stimulation and correlate with ELISA antibody measurement in Kawasaki disease. Clin Exp Immunol 1994;98: 264–9.

34. Sgonc R, Gruschwitz MS, Boeck G, et al. Endothelial cell apoptosis in systemic sclerosis is induced by antibody-dependent cell-mediated cytotoxicity via CD95. Arthritis Rheum 2000;43:2550–62.

35. Negi VS, Tripathy NK, Misra R, et al. Antiendothelial cell antibodies in sclero-derma correlate with severe digital ischemia and pulmonary arterial hyperten-sion. J Rheumatol 1998;25:462–6.

36. Song J, Park YB, Lee WK, et al. Clinical associations of anti-endothelial cell anti-bodies in patients with systemic lupus erythematosus. Rheumatol Int 2000;20:1–7.

37. Chan TM, Cheng IK. A prospective study on anti-endothelial cell antibodies in pa-tients with systemic lupus erythematosus. Clin Immunol Immunopathol 1996;78: 41–6.

38. Navarro M, Cervera R, Font J, et al. Anti-endothelial cell antibodies in systemic autoimmune diseases: prevalence and clinical significance. Lupus 1997;6:521–6.

39. Liu XD, Guo SY, Yang LL, et al. Anti-endothelial cell antibodies in connective tissue diseases associated with pulmonary arterial hypertension. J Thorac Dis 2014;6:497–502.

40. Tian W, Jiang X, Tamosiuniene R, et al. Blocking macrophage leukotriene b4 pre-vents endothelial injury and reverses pulmonary hypertension. Sci Transl Med 2013;5:200ra117.

41. van Bon L, Affandi AJ, Broen J, et al. Proteome-wide analysis and CXCL4 as a biomarker in systemic sclerosis. N Engl J Med 2014;370:433–43.

42. Wang Y, Kahaleh B. Epigenetic repression of bone morphogenetic protein recep-tor II expression in scleroderma. J Cell Mol Med 2013;17:1291–9.

43. Satoh M, Krzyszczak ME, Li Y, et al. Frequent coexistence of anti-topoisomerase I and anti-U1RNP autoantibodies in African American patients associated with mild skin involvement: a retrospective clinical study. Arthritis Res Ther 2011;13:R73.

44. Fredi M, Cavazzana I, Quinzanini M, et al. Rare autoantibodies to cellular anti-gens in systemic lupus erythematosus. Lupus 2014. [Epub ahead of print].

45. Okawa-Takatsuji M, Aotsuka S, Uwatoko S, et al. Increase of cytokine production by pulmonary artery endothelial cells induced by supernatants from monocytes stimulated with autoantibodies against U1-ribonucleoprotein. Clin Exp Rheumatol 1999;17:705–12.

46. Steen V, Medsger TA Jr. Predictors of isolated pulmonary hypertension in patients with systemic sclerosis and limited cutaneous involvement. Arthritis Rheum 2003; 48:516–22.

47. Stupi AM, Steen VD, Owens GR, et al. Pulmonary hypertension in the CREST syndrome variant of systemic sclerosis. Arthritis Rheum 1986;29:515–24.

48. Allanore Y, Borderie D, Avouac J, et al. High N-terminal pro-brain natriuretic peptide levels and low diffusing capacity for carbon monoxide as independent predictors of the occurrence of precapillary pulmonary arterial hypertension in patients with systemic sclerosis. Arthritis Rheum 2008;58:284–91.

49. Shah AA, Chung SE, Wigley FM, et al. Changes in estimated right ventricular systolic pressure predict mortality and pulmonary hypertension in a cohort of scleroderma patients. Ann Rheum Dis 2013;72:1136–40.

50. Valerio CJ, Schreiber BE, Handler CE, et al. Borderline mean pulmonary artery pressure in patients with systemic sclerosis: transpulmonary gradient predicts risk of developing pulmonary hypertension. Arthritis Rheum 2013;65:1074–84.
51. Heresi GA, Minai OA, Tonelli AR, et al. Clinical characterization and survival of patients with borderline elevation in pulmonary artery pressure. Pulm Circ 2013;3:916–25.
52. Yaqub A, Chung L. Epidemiology and risk factors for pulmonary hypertension in systemic sclerosis. Curr Rheumatol Rep 2013;15:302.
53. Gourh P, Arnett FC, Assassi S, et al. Plasma cytokine profiles in systemic sclerosis: associations with autoantibody subsets and clinical manifestations. Arthritis Res Ther 2009;11:R147.
54. Kollert F, Christoph S, Probst C, et al. Soluble CD90 as a potential marker of pulmonary involvement in systemic sclerosis. Arthritis Care Res 2013;65:281–7.
55. Fois E, Le Guern V, Dupuy A, et al. Noninvasive assessment of systolic pulmonary artery pressure in systemic lupus erythematosus: retrospective analysis of 93 patients. Clin Exp Rheumatol 2010;28:836–41.
56. Prabu A, Patel K, Yee CS, et al. Prevalence and risk factors for pulmonary arterial hypertension in patients with lupus. Rheumatology 2009;48:1506–11.
57. Thakkar V, Stevens WM, Moore OA, et al. Performance of screening algorithms in systemic sclerosis-related pulmonary arterial hypertension: a systematic review. Intern Med J 2013;43:751–60.
58. Saukkonen K, Tan TC, Sharma A, et al. Case records of the Massachusetts General Hospital. Case 9-2014. A 34-year-old woman with increasing dyspnea. N Engl J Med 2014;370:1149–57.
59. Prete M, Fatone MC, Vacca A, et al. Severe pulmonary hypertension as the initial manifestation of systemic lupus erythematosus: a case report and review of the literature. Clin Exp Rheumatol 2014;32:267–74.
60. Kuwana M, Watanabe H, Matsuoka N, et al. Pulmonary arterial hypertension associated with connective tissue disease: meta-analysis of clinical trials. BMJ Open 2013;3(8):e003113.
61. Taichman DB, Ornelas J, Chung L, et al. Pharmacologic therapy for pulmonary arterial hypertension in adults: CHEST guideline and expert panel report. Chest 2014;146:449–75.
62. Olsson KM, Delcroix M, Ghofrani HA, et al. Anticoagulation and survival in pulmonary arterial hypertension: results from the Comparative, Prospective Registry of Newly Initiated Therapies for Pulmonary Hypertension (COMPERA). Circulation 2014;129:57–65.
63. Nikpour M, Stevens W, Proudman SM, et al. Should patients with systemic sclerosis-related pulmonary arterial hypertension be anticoagulated? Intern Med J 2013;43:599–603.
64. Sanchez O, Sitbon O, Jais X, et al. Immunosuppressive therapy in connective tissue diseases-associated pulmonary arterial hypertension. Chest 2006;130:182–9.
65. Miyamichi-Yamamoto S, Fukumoto Y, Sugimura K, et al. Intensive immunosuppressive therapy improves pulmonary hemodynamics and long-term prognosis in patients with pulmonary arterial hypertension associated with connective tissue disease. Circ J 2011;75:2668–74.
66. Jais X, Launay D, Yaici A, et al. Immunosuppressive therapy in lupus- and mixed connective tissue disease-associated pulmonary arterial hypertension: a retrospective analysis of twenty-three cases. Arthritis Rheum 2008;58:521–31.
67. Tanaka E, Harigai M, Tanaka M, et al. Pulmonary hypertension in systemic lupus erythematosus: evaluation of clinical characteristics and response to immunosuppressive treatment. J Rheumatol 2002;29:282–7.

68. Kato M, Kataoka H, Odani T, et al. The short-term role of corticosteroid therapy for pulmonary arterial hypertension associated with connective tissue diseases: report of five cases and a literature review. Lupus 2011;20:1047–56.
69. Suzuki C, Takahashi M, Morimoto H, et al. Mycophenolate mofetil attenuates pulmonary arterial hypertension in rats. Biochem Biophys Res Commun 2006;349: 781–8.
70. Zheng Y, Li M, Zhang Y, et al. The effects and mechanisms of mycophenolate mofetil on pulmonary arterial hypertension in rats. Rheumatol Int 2010;30:341–8.
71. Morelli S, Giordano M, De Marzio P, et al. Pulmonary arterial hypertension responsive to immunosuppressive therapy in systemic lupus erythematosus. Lupus 1993;2:367–9.
72. McGonagle D, Tan AL, Madden J, et al. Successful treatment of resistant scleroderma-associated interstitial lung disease with rituximab. Rheumatology 2008;47:552–3.
73. Braun-Moscovici Y, Butbul-Aviel Y, Guralnik L, et al. Rituximab: rescue therapy in life-threatening complications or refractory autoimmune diseases: a single center experience. Rheumatol Int 2013;33:1495–504.
74. Hennigan S, Channick RN, Silverman GJ. Rituximab treatment of pulmonary arterial hypertension associated with systemic lupus erythematosus: a case report. Lupus 2008;17:754–6.
75. Jordan S, Distler JH, Maurer B, et al. Effects and safety of rituximab in systemic sclerosis: an analysis from the European Scleroderma Trial and Research (EUSTAR) group. Ann Rheum Dis 2014. [Epub ahead of print].
76. Daoussis D, Liossis SN, Tsamandas AC, et al. Experience with rituximab in scleroderma: results from a 1-year, proof-of-principle study. Rheumatology 2010;49:271–80.
77. Steen VD, Medsger TA. Changes in causes of death in systemic sclerosis, 1972-2002. Ann Rheum Dis 2007;66:940–4.
78. Tyndall AJ, Bannert B, Vonk M, et al. Causes and risk factors for death in systemic sclerosis: a study from the EULAR Scleroderma Trials and Research (EUSTAR) database. Ann Rheum Dis 2010;69:1809–15.
79. Chung L, Farber HW, Benza R, et al. Unique predictors of mortality in patients with pulmonary arterial hypertension associated with systemic sclerosis in the reveal registry. Chest 2014;146:1494–504.
80. Launay D, Sitbon O, Hachulla E, et al. Survival in systemic sclerosis-associated pulmonary arterial hypertension in the modern management era. Ann Rheum Dis 2013;72:1940–6.
81. Lefevre G, Dauchot L, Hachulla E, et al. Survival and prognostic factors in systemic sclerosis-associated pulmonary hypertension: a systematic review and meta-analysis. Arthritis Rheum 2013;65:2412–23.
82. Chung L, Domsic RT, Lingala B, et al. Survival and predictors of mortality in systemic sclerosis-associated pulmonary arterial hypertension: outcomes from the pulmonary hypertension assessment and recognition of outcomes in scleroderma registry. Arthritis Care Res 2014;66:489–95.
83. Chung SM, Lee CK, Lee EY, et al. Clinical aspects of pulmonary hypertension in patients with systemic lupus erythematosus and in patients with idiopathic pulmonary arterial hypertension. Clin Rheumatol 2006;25:866–72.
84. Launay D, Hachulla E, Hatron PY, et al. Pulmonary arterial hypertension: a rare complication of primary Sjogren syndrome: report of 9 new cases and review of the literature. Medicine 2007;86:299–315.

# Pulmonary Vasculitis

Lindsay Lally, MD*, Robert F. Spiera, MD

## KEYWORDS

- Diffuse alveolar hemorrhage • ANCA-associated vasculitis
- Granulomatosis with polyangiitis (Wegener) • Microscopic polyangiitis
- Antiphospholipid syndrome • Antiglomerular basement membrane disease
- Takayasu arteritis • Behçet syndrome

## KEY POINTS

- Pulmonary vasculitis most frequently occurs in the context of antineutrophil cytoplasmic antibody (ANCA)–associated vasculitis.
- In these disorders, pulmonary capillaritis with diffuse alveolar hemorrhage is the most common manifestation of small-vessel pulmonary vasculitis.
- Treatment of ANCA-associated vasculitis should be tailored to disease severity; diffuse alveolar hemorrhage represents a severe disease manifestation and warrants aggressive induction therapy.
- Pulmonary artery involvement in large vessel vasculitis such as Behçet syndrome and Takayasu arteritis may present as aneurysmal, thrombotic, or stenotic disease.

## INTRODUCTION

Systemic vasculitis refers to a clinicopathologically heterogeneous group of diseases classified most commonly by the size of the inflamed vessels and the organ systems affected. Pulmonary vasculitis encompasses inflammation in the pulmonary vasculature, with involved vessels varying in caliber from large elastic arteries to capillaries. Small pulmonary capillaries are the vessels most commonly involved in vasculitis affecting the lung.[1] The antineutrophil cytoplasmic antibody (ANCA)–associated vasculitides (AAVs), which include granulomatosis with polyangiitis (GPA, formerly Wegener granulomatosis), microscopic polyangiitis (MPA), and eosinophilic granulomatosis with polyangiitis (EGPA, formerly Churg-Strauss syndrome), are the small-vessel vasculitides in which pulmonary vasculitis is most frequently observed and

Disclosure Statement: The authors have nothing to disclose.
Division of Rheumatology, Hospital for Special Surgery, 535 East 70th Street, New York, NY 10021, USA
* Corresponding author.
E-mail address: lallyl@hss.edu

are the major focus of this article. Vasculitic involvement of the large pulmonary vessels, as may occur in Behçet syndrome and Takayasu arteritis (TA), is also discussed.

## SMALL-VESSEL VASCULITIS
### Diagnosis

#### Clinical presentation and physical examination
Although vasculitis of small pulmonary capillaries is the most common pathologic manifestation of pulmonary vasculitis, the clinical presentation is highly variable. Capillaritis and resultant destruction of the capillary-alveolar basement membrane leads to diffuse alveolar hemorrhage (DAH), characterized by extravasation of red blood cells into the alveolar spaces. A wide-spectrum of clinical signs and symptoms are associated with DAH; patients may be asymptomatic at presentation or present with acute respiratory failure. Symptoms usually arise over the course of several days, although more subacute presentations can occur. Most patients experience hemoptysis, although approximately one-third of patients with DAH do not report this condition at presentation.[2] Cough, fever, and dyspnea are other frequently occurring presenting manifestations. Similar to the presenting symptoms, physical examination findings in patients with DAH are typically nonspecific. Pulmonary auscultation may reveal decreased breath sounds or inspiratory crackles. Because DAH is the common denominator of many disease states injuring the pulmonary capillaries, specific clinical manifestations or examination findings suggestive of an underlying systemic disorder are discussed.

#### Laboratory findings
Anemia or a serially decreasing hemoglobin measurement is the most common laboratory finding in DAH, reflecting the accumulation of red blood cells in the alveolar spaces.[2] Leukocytosis or elevated inflammatory markers may be present, especially if the patient has an underlying systemic vasculitis. A retrospective analysis of almost 100 patients hospitalized for an initial episode of DAH suggested that a plasma lactate dehydrogenase (LDH) level greater than 2 times the upper limit of normal was an independent risk factor for in-hospital mortality.[3] In many cases, DAH is present as part of a pulmonary-renal syndrome with concurrent glomerular disease; thus, urinalysis may reveal elevated serum creatinine or active urine sediment levels. Specific serologic tests and detectable autoantibodies, which can be helpful in diagnosis, are highlighted in the discussion of the individual disease entities.

#### Radiology
Demonstration of bilateral air-space consolidation or opacities is the radiographic hallmark of DAH. Patchy, bilateral pulmonary infiltrates may be present on chest radiograph. Because the chest radiograph may be normal in DAH, a high-resolution computed tomography (CT) scan of the chest is recommended in patients with suspected DAH.[4] Chest CT often demonstrates ground glass opacities (GGOs) and can simultaneously rule out other causes of pulmonary hemorrhage, such as bronchiectasis or endobronchial tumor, in a patient with hemoptysis. In DAH, GGOs are often diffuse and bilateral; however, in approximately one-quarter of patients, the opacification is restricted to dependent areas of the lower lobes.[5] Imaging may lag behind clinical improvement and may take days to weeks to resolve after cessation of acute bleeding into the alveolar space. Following acute DAH, a radiographic pattern of septal thickening, known as crazy-paving, can occur, although, like GGO, this pattern is not specific for capillaritis or DAH.[6] Recurrent DAH can result in the development of pulmonary fibrosis, which is also readily apparent on high-resolution chest CT.

*Bronchoalveolar lavage*

Bronchoscopy accompanied by bronchoalveolar lavage (BAL) can confirm the diagnosis of DAH, which is particularly useful given the nonspecific clinical, laboratory, and radiographic presentation of DAH. Increasingly bloody return from serial BAL aliquots confirms acute alveolar hemorrhage. The presence of hemosiderin-laden macrophages on iron staining of the BAL fluid also supports DAH if more than 20% of the alveolar macrophages demonstrate iron staining. An additional advantage of BAL is the ability to concurrently rule out infection. Although BAL is useful in confirming hemorrhage, it has limited specificity in determining the underlying cause of DAH. Furthermore, BAL can fail to identify bleeding in some patients with DAH, most likely because of sampling error.

*Histopathology*

Guided-tissue biopsy from an affected organ is recommended to histologically confirm the diagnosis of small-vessel vasculitis whenever possible.[7] In the lung, targeted biopsy of radiographically abnormal lung parenchyma via either a thoracoscopic or open lung biopsy provides a high yield for diagnosis of small vessel vasculitis. Conversely, the efficacy of transbronchial biopsy in establishing the diagnosis of pulmonary vasculitis is less than 10%.[8] In a cohort of patients presenting with DAH who underwent open lung biopsy, capillaritis was documented in 88% of cases with a diagnosis of AAV or necrotizing small vessel vasculitis in 14 of 35 cases.[9] Neutrophilic aggregates interspersed within areas of hemorrhage and leukocytoclasia are seen in capillaritis. Histopathologic data must be interpreted in the context of known clinical and serologic data, and a final diagnosis can be further supported by immunofluorescence and with incorporation of other tissue histopathology if available.

## Differential Diagnosis

DAH can result from a variety of insults to the lung including autoimmune, infectious, neoplastic and toxic causes.[10,11] Broadly, DAH can be divided into immune-mediated and non–immune-mediated causes (**Box 1**). This distinction has critical initial management implications, because immune-mediated processes usually accompany systemic disease and warrant prompt administration of immunosuppressive medications, typically beginning with corticosteroids. A thorough history, including review of systems, past medical history, travel and exposure history, and drug use (including both prescription medications and illicit drugs), is helpful in identifying an underlying cause of DAH. Patients with immune-mediated DAH are more likely to report constitutional symptoms and arthritis and have evidence of renal involvement at presentation.[12] Frequently encountered immune-mediated causes of pulmonary capillaritis are discussed later; this article does not include a discussion of DAH in systemic lupus erythematosus or rheumatoid arthritis, because pulmonary involvement in these disorders is discussed elsewhere in this issue.

*ANCA-associated vasculitides*

The AAVs, encompassing GPA, MPA, and EGPA, are a heterogeneous group of necrotizing small vessel vasculitides with a predilection for the lung and kidney. As a group, these diseases account for the major cause of vasculitis affecting the lung. With the goal of redefining the vasculitic syndromes with nomenclature reflective of the underlying pathogenesis, pathologic conditions, and clinical characteristics, the 2012 Chapel Hill Consensus Conference eliminated eponyms from the AAV nomenclature.[13] In this revised classification system, the presence of granulomatous inflammation in the respiratory tract is the fundamental difference between GPA and MPA,

---

**Box 1**
**Selected causes of diffuse alveolar hemorrhage**

*Immune-mediated*

Systemic vasculitis

  ANCA-associated vasculitis

    Granulomatosis with polyangiitis

    Microscopic polyangiitis

    Eosinophilic granulomatosis with polyangiitis

    Drug-induced ANCA-associated vasculitis

  IgA vasculitis/Henoch-Schönlein purpura

  Cryoglobulinemic vasculitis

  Behçet syndrome

Connective tissue disease

    Antiglomerular basement membrane disease/Goodpasture syndrome

    Antiphospholipid syndrome

    Systemic lupus erythematosus

    Rheumatoid arthritis

Other

    Stem cell transplantation

    Lung transplant rejection

*Non–immune-mediated*

Infection

Congestive heart failure

Acute respiratory distress syndrome

Mitral stenosis/valvular heart disease

Drug-induced disease

Coagulopathy/anticoagulant use

Pulmonary hemosiderosis

---

whereas the presence of eosinophilia with granulomatous inflammation is the distinguishing feature of EGPA (formerly Churg-Strauss syndrome).

As the name implies, this group of systemic vasculitides share an association with serologically detectable ANCAs. Circulating ANCAs with different immunofluorescence patterns and antigen specificities characterize GPA and MPA and are an important diagnostic tool in these diseases. A perinuclear (p-ANCA) or cytoplasmic (c-ANCA) pattern may be seen on indirect immunofluorescence. A positive immunofluorescence pattern should be followed up with an enzyme-linked immunosorbent assay (ELISA) for ANCAs specifically directed against proteinase-3 (PR3) or myeloperoxidase (MPO), which are associated with GPA and MPA, respectively, in greater than 80% of cases.[14,15] Only approximately half of patients with EGPA have detectable ANCAs; when ANCA positivity is seen in EGPA, ANCAs are directed against MPO 75% of the time.[16] ANCA pattern on immunofluorescence and ELISA specificity must be interpreted together, because only combinations of c-ANCA with PR3 or p-ANCA with MPO have a high positive predictive value for GPA or MPA diagnosis. Certain drugs, infections, and malignancies can cause ANCA positivity; thus, the diagnostic utility of ANCAs depends on the clinical setting in which testing occurs. In patients presenting with DAH or a pulmonary-renal syndrome, ANCA positivity is highly suggestive of AAV and can help elucidate the underlying cause of DAH.

Some form of pulmonary involvement occurs in most patients with AAV, and may range from asymptomatic pulmonary nodules to fulminant respiratory failure, as may occur in approximately 25% of patients with AAV and DAH.[17] Approximately 85% of patients with GPA and MPA will have pulmonary involvement during their disease course,[18] whereas asthma is the hallmark feature of EGPA, occurring in more than 90% of patients.[19] Although overlap exists, those with GPA are more likely to develop nodules or cavitary lung disease, whereas interstitial disease and pulmonary fibrosis occur more frequently in MPA (**Table 1**). Furthermore, pulmonary involvement at disease presentation may predict long-term development of damage, with one study suggesting that those with pulmonary disease at AAV diagnosis had significantly higher damage scores at 2 years than those without pulmonary disease at presentation, and had an increased likelihood of developing pulmonary fibrosis.[20] An estimated 25% of those with DAH at presentation will have persistent abnormalities on pulmonary function testing.[21]

A recent systematic review analyzed more than 200 patients with AAV who had DAH with a reported incidence of 8% to 36%[17]; DAH occurred most frequently in those with MPA, who constituted 52% of the cohort, whereas DAH was rare in EGPA (6%). Other cohorts of patients with AAV and DAH have been more enriched for GPA than MPA.[22] DAH also occurs in children with AAV, with a reported incidence of 40% in one small series of pediatric patients with MPA.[23]

Extrapulmonary disease often accompanies pulmonary vasculitis in AAV and should be evaluated for in patients with suspected AAV and DAH. Fevers, arthralgia/arthritis, myalgia, and weight loss related to underlying systemic vasculitis often occur with DAH. Granulomatous involvement of the otolaryngologic system, including rhinosinusitis, serous otitis, and subglottic inflammation, occurs in greater than 90% of patients with GPA and is commonly a feature at disease presentation.[18] As such, a focused history and examination can gauge disease activity in this domain and, in conjunction with other clinical and serologic data, can support the diagnosis of GPA. Thorough assessment for all organ systems involved in these systemic disorders is crucial for determination of disease activity and stratification of disease severity.

Renal disease in the form of rapidly progressive glomerulonephritis accompanies DAH in most patients with AAV[17,21,22,24]; thus, assessing for renal involvement with urinalysis, serum creatinine measurement, and possibly kidney biopsy, when indicated, can help confirm an AAV diagnosis and provide information for disease stratification and prognosis.[25] Unlike renal involvement, some studies suggest that DAH alone is not predictive of poor outcome or increased mortality,[22] although others have found

| Table 1 | |
|---|---|
| **Distinguishing pulmonary features in ANCA-associated vasculitides** | |
| **AAV Subtype** | **Distinguishing Pulmonary Features** |
| GPA | Nodules, cavities, endobronchial lesions |
| MPA | Interstitial lung disease, fibrosis |
| EGPA | Asthma, infiltrates, eosinophilic pleural effusions |

that DAH increased the relative risk of death by a factor of 8 and is thus a strong predictor of early mortality in AAV.[17] Additional poor prognostic factors that have been identified in patients with AAV with pulmonary vasculitis include intensive care unit admission and mechanical ventilation.[26]

In approaching AAV therapy, a few critical treatment principles guide patient management. First, patients should be stratified by disease severity, with treatment tailored to severity of disease. Severe disease, defined as life- or organ-threatening manifestations, includes features such as DAH, rapidly progressive glomerulonephritis, mesenteric ischemia, scleritis, and nervous system involvement, and typically requires more aggressive therapy.[27] Limited disease, which encompasses all non–life- or organ-threatening manifestations, including mild renal or granulomatous or nodular pulmonary disease, may not require immunosuppression that is as potent. Similarly, disease flares or relapses should be characterized as limited or severe based on organ systems involved, and this distinction is considered when choosing therapy.

Historically, AAV was treated with cyclophosphamide-based regimens after the recognition that a regimen of daily oral cyclophosphamide and high-dose corticosteroids was effective for inducing remission in most patients, which transformed GPA and MPA from a uniformly fatal disease to a chronic relapsing disease with a dramatically reduced mortality of 25% at 5 years.[28] Subsequent appreciation of the toxicity associated with long-term cyclophosphamide use[18] led to the search for therapeutic regimens that minimized and/or avoided cyclophosphamide exposure. Therefore, treatment of AAV is divided into therapy aimed at inducing remission followed by use of remission-maintenance agents.

Corticosteroids remain part of all induction regimens in active or relapsing disease and are usually tapered once remission is attained. Some patients are maintained on low-dose corticosteroids during the maintenance period, although at most centers, the goal is complete discontinuation after remission induction. The optimal tapering regimen and duration of glucocorticoid treatment is not established.

As mentioned previously, cyclophosphamide in combination with high-dose corticosteroids was long considered the standard of care for remission-induction therapy in patients with severe AAV. Complete remission is attainable in greater than 75% of patients treated with oral cyclophosphamide at doses of 2 mg/kg/d (with dose reductions made for older age and renal insufficiency). Use of pulsed intravenous cyclophosphamide (15 mg/kg every 2–3 weeks) has comparable efficacy to oral cyclophosphamide, with the advantage of lower cumulative cyclophosphamide doses.[29] However, those treated with intravenous cyclophosphamide may have higher relapse rates than those treated with the oral formulation.[30] Thus, cyclophosphamide regimens are similar in their ability to induce remission, with possibly higher relapse rates associated with intravenous cyclophosphamide, which must be balanced with the higher rates of leukopenia and potential infection associated with daily oral regimens.

Targeting of B cells with rituximab, the monoclonal anti-CD20 antibody, has been demonstrated to be an effective therapy for remission induction in severe AAV.[31,32] Two randomized trials including patients with both newly diagnosed and relapsing severe AAV demonstrated that rituximab was noninferior to cyclophosphamide for remission induction. In the double-blind, double-dummy Rituximab in ANCA-Associated Vasculitis (RAVE) trial, a single course of rituximab (375 mg/m$^2$ weekly for 4 weeks) was compared with cyclophosphamide followed by azathioprine in 197 patients with AAV; all patients received high-dose intravenous corticosteroids at the beginning of the induction regimen. Patients with a serum creatinine level greater than 4 mg/dL or alveolar hemorrhage requiring mechanical ventilatory support were excluded from RAVE. The criteria for noninferiority were met, with 64% of patients receiving rituximab versus 53% of those receiving cyclophosphamide achieving steroid-free disease remission at 6 months, with similar rates of flare and serious adverse events noted in both groups. Published concurrent to RAVE, the Rituximab Versus Cyclophosphamide in ANCA-Associated Renal Vasculitis (RITUXVAS) study was an open-label trial in patients with newly diagnosed AAV with renal involvement. Patients were randomized 3:1 to receive rituximab (375 mg/m$^2$ weekly for 4 weeks) plus 2 doses of intravenous cyclophosphamide or pulse intravenous cyclophosphamide alone along with background corticosteroids in both groups. At 12 months, 76% of patients in the rituximab/cyclophosphamide group and 82% of patients in the cyclophosphamide-only group had achieved sustained remission. Although rituximab-only regimens have not been studied extensively in patients with severe DAH and respiratory failure, a combination of rituximab and cyclophosphamide for critically ill patients with AAV may be beneficial.[33] Local pulmonary administration of activated factor VII has been used successfully to treat DAH.[34] Although factor VII use has been reported to provide local control of pulmonary hemorrhage in patients with AAV.[35] its use cannot supplant systemic therapy aimed at controlling the underlying disease.

Removal of the circulating pathogenic ANCAs with plasma exchange has been used as adjunctive therapy in patients with severe AAV, including those with active glomerulonephritis and DAH. Used in conjunction with standard induction therapy, plasma exchange may improve renal recovery in patients dependent on dialysis and those with severe renal disease but does not seem to improve overall survival.[36,37] No controlled trials of patients with AAV and DAH treated with plasma exchange have been reported, although retrospective data suggest that this therapy may provide benefit.[38] An international randomized controlled study to evaluate the efficacy of plasma exchange in patients with AAV, DAH, and/or severe renal disease is ongoing.[39]

In patients with limited disease, which by definition can include patients with pulmonary involvement whose oxygen saturation by pulse oximetry is greater than 92% or room air partial pressure of oxygen is greater than 70 mm Hg,[27] cyclophosphamide-free induction regimens are commonly used. Despite this definition, when alveolar hemorrhage is present, disease is typically categorized as serious, requiring more aggressive immunosuppressive therapy. Methotrexate can be used to induce remission in limited AAV. An open-label trial comparing methotrexate with cyclophosphamide randomized patients with newly diagnosed AAV and limited disease (including mild renal and pulmonary involvement) to either methotrexate, 15 to 25 mg weekly or oral cyclophosphamide.[40] The primary end point of remission at 6 months was achieved in 90% of methotrexate-treated patients and 94% of cyclophosphamide-treated patients, although patients on methotrexate took a longer time to achieve remission and had higher rates of relapse at 18 months, most of which occurred after therapy was tapered off.[41]

Most patients who receive cyclophosphamide induction therapy are switched to an alternative maintenance therapy after 3 to 6 months, depending on clinical response. Azathioprine and methotrexate are the principal conventional immunosuppressive agents used for remission maintenance in AAV. The efficacy and safety of azathioprine for maintenance were demonstrated in a study in which patients who had achieved remission on oral cyclophosphamide were randomized to continue treatment with cyclophosphamide at a lower dose or to switch to azathioprine.[42] No difference was seen in relapse rates at 18 months between the 2 treatment groups, nor was a difference in adverse events observed. Methotrexate and azathioprine were also compared in a head-to-head maintenance trial, in which the primary end point was adverse events requiring discontinuation of therapy.[43] Rates of adverse events and relapse were similar between those receiving methotrexate and those taking azathioprine; thus, methotrexate and azathioprine seem to be comparably efficacious and safe maintenance agents in AAV. Conversely, when mycophenolate mofetil (MMF) was compared with azathioprine for maintenance, relapse rates were higher in the MMF treatment arm, with a hazard ratio of 1.69, but no difference was seen in serious adverse events.[44] Because MMF is less efficacious than azathioprine in preventing relapse, it is not routinely used as a first-line maintenance therapy in AAV, although it may have a role in treating patients with refractory disease or those intolerant of other agents.

Rituximab is an also an effective maintenance therapy for AAV. A follow-up of RAVE reported that complete remission rates at 12 and 18 months were comparable in patients who had received a single course of rituximab and those who received cyclophosphamide followed by azathioprine maintenance.[45] These data suggest that, given the prolonged duration of its biological effects, a single course of rituximab has comparable safety and efficacy to continuous conventional immunosuppressive therapy in remission induction and maintenance out to 18 months. The optimal dose and frequency of rituximab maintenance therapy remain unknown. Some studies support the use of a preemptive strategy of rituximab retreatment every 6 months,[46,47] whereas other investigators advocate for utility in the combination of B lymphocyte reconstitution and ANCA level in predicting relapse, and base the retreatment decision on these laboratory parameters.[48] More definitive studies comparing these rituximab retreatment strategies and a head-to-head comparison of rituximab and azathioprine for maintenance are currently underway.

Once remission is induced and patients are on maintenance therapy, structured clinical assessments with urinalysis and basic laboratory tests should be performed regularly to monitor for new organ involvement, treatment response, and drug toxicity.[7] Relapse is common in AAV, especially after discontinuation of immunosuppression. The optimal duration of maintenance therapy is unknown. Relapse rates, which approach 55% in some cohorts, are highest in the first few years after diagnosis; thus, maintenance immunosuppression is generally continued for approximately 2 years in most patients.[49] Duration of maintenance therapy should be individualized and balance the individual risk of relapse with treatment morbidity. The main cause of death in the first year of AAV diagnosis is infection, accounting for 48% of deaths compared with 19% caused by active vasculitis, and therefore the risk of immunosuppression is not trivial.[28] Patients with AAV have been shown to have higher rates of *Pneumocystis jirovecii* pneumonia (PCP) than other patients with autoimmune disease on similar immunosuppressive regimens. Although no guidelines exist, PCP prophylaxis should be considered in all patients with AAV receiving induction therapy with either cyclophosphamide or rituximab. Vaccination is an important infection prevention strategy for patients with AAV. Although no disease-specific or medication-specific vaccination guidelines are available for patients with vasculitis, the Centers for Disease Control and Prevention guidelines for immunocompromised individuals can be applied to those on immunosuppressive treatment for AAV.[50]

### Antiphospholipid syndrome

Antiphospholipid syndrome (APS) is an autoimmune disease characterized by vascular thrombosis and/or pregnancy morbidity occurring in the presence of serologically detectable antiphospholipid antibodies (aPLs). aPLs, which are autoantibodies directed against phospholipid-binding plasma proteins, include lupus anticoagulant (LAC), anticardiolipin antibody, and anti–β2-glycoprotein I (aβ2GPI) and should be persistently positive when measured at least 12 weeks apart to meet criteria for APS.[51] APS may occur alone or in the setting of another autoimmune disease, most commonly systemic lupus erythematosus.

Although the most common clinical manifestations of APS are thrombosis and fetal loss, it is a multisystem disease with many noncriteria manifestations, including thrombocytopenia, skin ulcers, and nephropathy.[52] The pathogenic vascular lesions in APS are principally related to thrombosis or microangiopathy, and not inflammation, although vasculitis, such as capillaritis, may rarely be a component of APS.[53]

Pulmonary involvement with DAH is a rare but serious manifestation of APS.[54] DAH occurs more frequently in the catastrophic antiphospholipid syndrome (CAPS) than in classic APS.[55] The histopathologic pulmonary capillaritis in APS/CAPS is believed to be immune-mediated, with circulating aPLs implicated in the pathogenesis.[56] In the largest reported series of primary APS-associated DAH, which described 18 patients, histologic evidence of capillaritis was noted in all 3 patients who underwent surgical lung biopsy.[57] Bronchial alveolar lavage has shown that neutrophilia and neutrophils are often present in the alveolar space on biopsy specimens even if capillaritis is not seen.[58] These inflammatory pathologic findings in APS-associated DAH occur in the absence of thrombosis; thus, DAH is considered to be a nonthrombotic manifestation of APS.

The presumed inflammatory nature of DAH in APS has important therapeutic implications. Experts recommend prompt initial treatment of DAH with high-dose corticosteroids and temporary cessation of anticoagulation.[54,57] Additional immunosuppression is often needed, because recurrence and mortality are common. No controlled or prospective data are available to guide treatment of APS-related DAH; however, borrowing from the treatment of capillaritis in AAV, cyclophosphamide or rituximab are often the first-line agents used. In a recent retrospective series from the Mayo Clinic of 18 patients with primary APS-associated DAH, complete remission was achieved in 3 of 7 patients treated with cyclophosphamide and 5 of 8 patients treated with a rituximab-based regimen, whereas uncontrolled disease was observed in patients treated with azathioprine, MMF, intravenous immunoglobulin, or plasmapheresis.[57]

### Antiglomerular basement membrane antibody disease

Antiglomerular basement membrane antibody disease (anti-GBM disease), also known as Goodpasture disease, is an immune complex–mediated small vessel vasculitis.[13] The cause of anti-GBM disease is unknown, but genetic factors affect susceptibility and environmental factors are associated with the disease.[59] The hallmark of disease is detectable anti-GBM antibodies, which are directed against and ultimately bind to the noncollagenous-I domain of type IV collagen in the basement membrane.[60] Anti-GBM antibodies can be detected in the sera via an ELISA-based assay or can be demonstrated histologically in biopsy specimens of affected tissue.

Acute renal failure from rapidly progressive crescentic glomerulonephritis is the most common presenting feature of anti-GBM disease. Renal biopsy, which will demonstrate linear deposits of IgG under immunofluorescence, is more sensitive than serology in confirming the diagnosis and also provides prognostic information.[61] Anti-GBM disease can present as pulmonary-renal syndrome with DAH accompanying crescentic glomerulonephritis in approximately 50% of cases.[62–64] Patients presenting with DAH in the absence of frank renal involvement have a better prognosis and, according to some cohorts, are more likely to be younger than those with renal involvement.[62,65] Predominant pulmonary involvement is often associated with smoking, prior exposure to inhaled toxins, or pulmonary infection. Some researchers have speculated that these exposures may trigger disease by damaging the pulmonary endothelium, which can expose the basement membrane and allow it to serve as an antigenic stimulus for anti-GBM antibody production and/or a binding target for circulating antibodies.

Renal involvement and risk for rapid progression to end-stage renal disease drives therapy in anti-GBM disease. High serum creatinine levels at baseline and percentage of crescents on renal biopsy confer a poor prognosis, highlighting the importance of early diagnosis and treatment, because most patients who require hemodialysis at presentation remain dialysis-dependent.[66] "Triple therapy" is considered the gold standard for anti-GBM disease treatment, with a regimen including corticosteroids, immunosuppressives, and plasmapheresis,[67] resulting in a 1-year survival rate approaching 90%.

Plasmapheresis to remove the pathogenic anti-GBM antibody is essential to the management of anti-GBM disease. Plasmapheresis is typically prescribed daily for 10 to 14 days or until anti-GBM antibodies are no longer detectable; albumin is the usual replacement fluid for exchanges but fresh frozen plasma can be used instead to replace coagulation factors in patients with active DAH.[68]

In a small controlled trial that randomized patients to receive corticosteroids with or without plasma exchange,[69] only 2 of 8 patients receiving plasma exchange developed end-stage renal disease, compared with 6 of 9 patients who received only immunosuppressives. Although this study was underpowered and therefore a significant result was not reached, it shifted the treatment paradigm to include plasmapheresis in most cases of anti-GBM disease. Use of plasmapheresis in patients who are already dialysis-dependent is debated, because longitudinal studies suggest a very low probability (<10%) for return of renal function in these patients.[65] The decision to use plasmapheresis in these patients should take into account the duration of renal failure and prognostic features on renal biopsy.

Similar to other vasculitic syndromes, the cornerstone of treatment is a regimen that includes high-dose corticosteroids and cyclophosphamide. Most of the experience using cyclophosphamide in anti-GBM disease is with the oral formulation given at a dosage of 2 mg/kg/d, again with adjustments made for creatinine clearance and older age.[65] Corticosteroids at a dose of 1 mg/kg are usually administered initially, with a slow tapering over the next several months pending the patient's clinical response. The successful use of rituximab either alone or in combination with cyclophosphamide has been reported.[70] Unlike in AAV, anti-GBM titers can correlate with disease activity and be used to determine duration of therapy; experts recommend continuation of steroids and maintenance therapy with azathioprine if anti-GBM titers remain elevated after 4 months of cyclophosphamide, whereas those with persistently negative titers on serial monitoring do not typically require maintenance medications.

A subset of patients have both anti-GBM and ANCA. This "double positivity" may occur in approximately 20% to 30% of patients with anti-GBM disease. When present, the ANCA specificity is usually directed against MPO. These patients tend to have more extrarenal involvement than those with pure anti-GBM disease, whereas clinically and histologically, their renal disease parallels that of other patients with anti-GBM disease.[71] Although some studies have suggested increased relapse rates and mortality in double-positive patients,[72] other cohorts show that renal survival in double-positive patients is similar to that in other patients with anti-GBM positivity and considerably worse than in those with only MPO positivity.[73]

## LARGE VESSEL VASCULITIS

Vasculitic involvement of the large pulmonary arteries can cause aneurysmal changes, stenosis, or occlusion. Isolated pulmonary artery vasculitis is rare and typically occurs in the context of a systemic vasculitis, such as Behçet's syndrome or TA.

### Behçet Syndrome

Behçet syndrome is classified as a variable-vessel vasculitis, meaning small, medium, or large vessels in the arterial or venous system can be involved in the inflammatory process, although large vessel disease is most common. Recurrent oral and genital ulcers are a hallmark of Behçet syndrome. Other manifestations can include skin lesions, arthritis, uveitis, gastrointestinal ulceration, and vascular involvement.

Pulmonary artery aneurysms (PAAs) and/or thrombosis are severe manifestations of Behçet syndrome. Although PAAs are a rare manifestation of Behçet syndrome, occurring in less than 10% of patients, they are an independent risk factor for and important contributor to mortality.[74] Though Behçet syndrome has no gender predilection, pulmonary vascular involvement occurs almost exclusively in male patients. In a series of 47 patients with Behçet syndrome and pulmonary artery involvement, 34 had PAA, whereas 8 had PAA with concurrent pulmonary artery thrombosis and 13 had isolated pulmonary artery thrombosis.[75] Concurrent abnormalities in multiple branches of the pulmonary artery is a usual finding radiographically.

Patients with Behçet syndrome with pulmonary artery involvement most commonly present with hemoptysis; fever, dyspnea, cough, and pleuritic chest pain are also frequent presenting symptoms. Pulmonary artery involvement in Behçet syndrome can be diagnosed with several imaging techniques, including CT angiography, MR angiography and fluorodeoxyglucose F 18/PET scanning.[76–78] Extrapulmonary disease usually accompanies PAA. Pulmonary arterial disease is associated with peripheral vascular disease in approximately 75% of patients, typically presenting as thrombophlebitis with superficial or deep vein thrombosis.[79] Thrombi in Behçet syndrome are usually surrounded by an inflammatory infiltrate. Management of venous thrombosis in Behçet syndrome is controversial, with some experts supporting treatment with immunosuppression rather than anticoagulation and others suggesting a combination of immunosuppression with concurrent anticoagulation.[80]

Controlled studies of treatment for PAA in Behçet syndrome are lacking, although most series in the literature report a combination of high-dose corticosteroids with either cyclophosphamide, azathioprine, or infliximab.[74,81,82] Anticoagulation is sometimes used for patients with stenotic or occlusive disease. For refractory hemoptysis, surgical interventions such as endovascular embolization and even lobectomy have been reported.[83,84]

### Takayasu Arteritis

TA is a granulomatous large vessel vasculitis predominantly affecting the aorta and its major branches. TA preferentially affects women younger than 50 years. Prevalence estimates of pulmonary arteritis in TA vary between 15% and 60%, which may partly reflect the asymptomatic nature of pulmonary artery involvement in many patients.[85,86] Pulmonary arteritis usually occurs in conjunction with disease in other large vessels, but isolated pulmonary arteritis in TA has been reported.[87]

Presenting symptoms of pulmonary artery involvement in TA include dyspnea, cough, chest pain, and hemoptysis.[88] Pulmonary arterial hypertension is an important complication of pulmonary arteritis seen in patients with TA. Because the presenting signs and symptoms of pulmonary involvement in TA may be nonspecific or even absent, imaging plays an important role in diagnosis. In one series examining 15 asymptomatic patients with TA, 60% had evidence of pulmonary vascular involvement on noninvasive imaging using perfusion and ventilation lung scintigraphy.[89] CT angiography and MR angiography have largely supplanted conventional angiography in the assessment of pulmonary vascular disease, because of their noninvasive nature and ability to detect subtle changes in the vessel wall, which can help differentiate active disease from stenosis caused by previously damaged vasculature. The use of PET in assessment of aortic/large vessel disease in TA is an area of active investigation[90]; however, negative PET imaging results in patients with TA with known pulmonary artery involvement have been reported, with the hypothesized explanation that the diameter of the pulmonary arteries is less than the power of detection of PET.[91]

Treatment of pulmonary artery involvement follows the general treatment principles for TA, in that high-dose corticosteroids are typically the first-line agents.[92] Methotrexate or azathioprine is often used in conjunction with steroids. For refractory or life-threatening disease, cyclophosphamide has been used, although more recently, biologic agents such as infliximab, rituximab, or tocilizumab are often used as an alternative to cyclophosphamide.[93] Again, no controlled data or head-to-head comparisons on the use of these therapies in TA are available. Relapses are common when immunosuppression is tapered, and the optimal duration of therapy is also unknown. Surgical therapies, including angioplasty, stenting, bypass, and even pulmonary artery replacement, have been reported to manage pulmonary artery stenosis in TA.[94,95] Generally, surgical interventions should only be undertaken once the disease is quiescent, and even then restenosis is common.

## SUMMARY

Many of the systemic vasculitides can cause inflammation of the pulmonary vasculature. Whether the small pulmonary capillaries or the pulmonary arteries are involved in the vasculitic process, presenting signs and symptoms may be nonspecific and a high index of suspicion is necessary to diagnose pulmonary vasculitis. Pulmonary vascular involvement usually represents a serious disease manifestation of systemic vasculitis requiring prompt treatment with corticosteroids and additional immunosuppressive agents.

## REFERENCES

1. Mark EJ, Ramirez JF. Pulmonary capillaritis and hemorrhage in patients with systemic vasculitis. Arch Pathol Lab Med 1985;109:413–8.
2. Collard HR, Schwarz MI. Diffuse alveolar hemorrhage. Clin Chest Med 2004;25: 583–92.
3. de Prost N, Parrot A, Picard C, et al. Diffuse alveolar haemorrhage: factors associated with in-hospital and long-term mortality. Eur Respir J 2010;35:1303–11.
4. Krause ML, Cartin-Ceba R, Specks U, et al. Update on diffuse alveolar hemorrhage and pulmonary vasculitis. Immunol Allergy Clin North Am 2012;32: 587–600.
5. Chung MP, Yi CA, Lee HY, et al. Imaging of pulmonary vasculitis. Radiology 2010; 255:322–41.
6. Spira D, Wirths S, Skowronski F, et al. Diffuse alveolar hemorrhage in patients with hematological malignancies: HRCT patterns of pulmonary involvement and disease course. Clin Imaging 2013;37:680–6.
7. Mukhtyar C, Guillevin L, Cid MC, et al, European Vasculitis Study Group. EULAR recommendations for management of primary small and medium vessel vasculitis. Ann Rheum Dis 2009;68:310–7.

8. Schnabel A, Holl-Ulrich K, Dalhoff K, et al. Efficacy of transbronchial biopsy in pulmonary vasculitides. Eur Respir J 1997;10:2738–43.

9. Travis WD, Colby TV, Lombard C, et al. A clinicopathologic study of 34 cases of diffuse pulmonary hemorrhage with lung biopsy confirmation. Am J Surg Pathol 1990;14:1112–25.

10. von Ranke FM, Zanetti G, Hochhegger B, et al. Infectious diseases causing diffuse alveolar hemorrhage in immunocompetent patients: a state-of-the-art review. Lung 2013;191:9–18.

11. Jin SM, Yim JJ, Yoo CG, et al. Aetiologies and outcomes of diffuse alveolar haemorrhage presenting as acute respiratory failure of uncertain cause. Respirology 2009;14:290–4.

12. de Prost N, Parrot A, Cuquemelle E, et al. Immune diffuse alveolar hemorrhage: a retrospective assessment of a diagnostic scale. Lung 2013;191:559–63.

13. Jennette JC, Falk RJ, Bacon PA, et al. 2012 revised International Chapel Hill Consensus Conference Nomenclature of Vasculitides. Arthritis Rheum 2013;65:1–11.

14. Guillevin L, Durand-Gasselin B, Cevallos R, et al. Microscopic polyangiitis: clinical and laboratory findings in eighty-five patients. Arthritis Rheum 1999;42:421–30.

15. Finkielman JD, Lee AS, Hummel AM, et al. ANCA are detectable in nearly all patients with active severe Wegener's granulomatosis. Am J Med 2007;120(7):9–14.

16. Sablé-Fourtassou R, Cohen P, Mahr A, et al. Antineutrophil cytoplasmic antibodies in the Churg-Strauss syndrome. Ann Intern Med 2005;143:632–8.

17. West S, Arulkumaran N, Ind PW, et al. Diffuse alveolar haemorrhage in ANCA-associated vasculitis. Intern Med 2013;52:5–13.

18. Hoffman GS, Kerr GS, Leavitt RY, et al. Wegener's granulomatosis: an analysis of 158 patients. Ann Intern Med 1992;116:488–98.

19. Comarmond C, Pagnoux C, Khellaf M, et al. Eosinophilic granulomatosis with polyangiitis (Churg-Strauss): clinical characteristics and long-term followup of the 383 patients enrolled in the French Vasculitis Study Group cohort. Arthritis Rheum 2013;65:270–81.

20. Hassan TM, Hassan AS, Igoe A, et al. Lung involvement at presentation predicts disease activity and permanent organ damage at 6, 12 and 24 months follow - up in ANCA - associated vasculitis. BMC Immunol 2014;15:20.

21. Lauque D, Cadranel J, Lazor R, et al. Microscopic polyangiitis with alveolar hemorrhage. A study of 29 cases and review of the literature. Groupe d'Etudes et de Recherche sur les Maladies "Orphelines" Pulmonaires (GERM"O"P). Medicine (Baltimore) 2000;79:222–33.

22. Kostianovsky A, Hauser T, Pagnoux C, et al. Alveolar haemorrhage in ANCA-associated vasculitides: 80 patients' features and prognostic factors. Clin Exp Rheumatol 2012;30:S77–82.

23. Ben Ameur S, Niaudet P, Baudouin V, et al. Lung manifestations in MPO-ANCA associated vasculitides in children. Pediatr Pulmonol 2014;49:285–90.

24. Lin Y, Zheng W, Tian X, et al. Antineutrophil cytoplasmic antibody-associated vasculitis complicated with diffuse alveolar hemorrhage: a study of 12 cases. J Clin Rheumatol 2009;15:341–4.

25. Ford SL, Polkinghorne KR, Longano A, et al. Histopathologic and clinical predictors of kidney outcomes in ANCA-associated vasculitis. Am J Kidney Dis 2014;63:227–35.

26. Holguin F, Ramadan B, Gal AA, et al. Prognostic factors for hospital mortality and ICU admission in patients with ANCA-related pulmonary vasculitis. Am J Med Sci 2008;336(4):321–6.

27. Stone JH, Wegener's Granulomatosis Etanercept Trial Research Group. Limited versus severe Wegener's granulomatosis: baseline data on patients in the Wegener's granulomatosis etanercept trial. Arthritis Rheum 2003;48:2299–309.

28. Flossmann O, Berden A, de Groot K, et al. Long-term patient survival in ANCA-associated vasculitis. Ann Rheum Dis 2011;70:488–94.

29. de Groot K, Harper L, Jayne DR, et al. Pulse versus daily oral cyclophosphamide for induction of remission in antineutrophil cytoplasmic antibody-associated vasculitis: a randomized trial. Ann Intern Med 2009;150:670–80.

30. Harper L, Morgan MD, Walsh M, et al. Pulse versus daily oral cyclophosphamide for induction of remission in ANCA-associated vasculitis: long-term follow-up. Ann Rheum Dis 2012;71:955–60.

31. Stone JH, Merkel PA, Spiera R, et al. Rituximab versus cyclophosphamide for ANCA-associated vasculitis. N Engl J Med 2010;363:221–32.

32. Jones RB, Tervaert JW, Hauser T, et al. Rituximab versus cyclophosphamide in ANCA-associated renal vasculitis. N Engl J Med 2010;363:211–20.

33. Baird EM, Lehman TJ, Worgall S. Combination therapy with rituximab and cyclophosphamide in the treatment of anti-neutrophil cytoplasmic antibodies (ANCA) positive pulmonary hemorrhage: case report. Pediatr Rheumatol Online J 2011; 9(1):33–6.

34. Heslet L, Nielsen JD, Nepper-Christensen S. Local pulmonary administration of factor VIIa (rFVIIa) in diffuse alveolar hemorrhage (DAH) - a review of a new treatment paradigm. Biologics 2012;6:37–46.

35. Dabar G, Harmouche C, Jammal M. Efficacy of recombinant activated factor VII in diffuse alveolar haemorrhage. Rev Mal Respir 2011;28:106–11.

36. Pusey CD, Rees AJ, Evans DJ, et al. Plasma exchange in focal necrotizing glomerulonephritis without anti-GBM antibodies. Kidney Int 1991;40:757–63.

37. Jayne DR, Gaskin G, Rasmussen N, et al. Randomized trial of plasma exchange or high-dosage methylprednisolone as adjunctive therapy for severe renal vasculitis. J Am Soc Nephrol 2007;18:2180–8.

38. Klemmer PJ, Chalermskulrat W, Reif MS, et al. Plasmapheresis therapy for diffuse alveolar hemorrhage in patients with small-vessel vasculitis. Am J Kidney Dis 2003;42:1149–52.

39. Walsh M, Merkel PA, Peh CA, et al. Plasma exchange and glucocorticoid dosing in the treatment of anti-neutrophil cytoplasm antibody associated vasculitis (PEX-IVAS): protocol for a randomized controlled trial. Trials 2013;14:73–6.

40. De Groot K, Rasmussen N, Bacon PA, et al. Randomized trial of cyclophosphamide versus methotrexate for induction of remission in early systemic antineutrophil cytoplasmic antibody-associated vasculitis. Arthritis Rheum 2005;52: 2461–89.

41. Faurschou M, Westman K, Rasmussen N, et al. Brief report: long-term outcome of a randomized clinical trial comparing methotrexate to cyclophosphamide for remission induction in early systemic antineutrophil cytoplasmic antibody-associated vasculitis. Arthritis Rheum 2012;34:3472–7.

42. Jayne D, Rasmussen N, Andrassy K, et al. A randomized trial of maintenance therapy for vasculitis associated with antineutrophil cytoplasmic autoantibodies. N Engl J Med 2003;349:36–44.

43. Pagnoux C, Mahr A, Hamidou MA, et al. Azathioprine or methotrexate maintenance for ANCA-associated vasculitis. N Engl J Med 2008;359:2790–803.

44. Hiemstra TF, Walsh M, Mahr A, et al. Mycophenolate mofetil vs azathioprine for remission maintenance in antineutrophil cytoplasmic antibody-associated vasculitis: a randomized controlled trial. JAMA 2010;304:2381–8.

45. Specks U, Merkel PA, Seo P, et al. Efficacy of remission-induction regimens for ANCA-associated vasculitis. N Engl J Med 2013;369:417–27.

46. Smith RM, Jones RB, Guerry M, et al. Rituximab for remission maintenance in relapsing antineutrophil cytoplasmic antibody-associated vasculitis. Arthritis Rheum 2012;64:3760–9.

47. Calich AL, Puéchal X, Pugnet G, et al. Rituximab for induction and maintenance therapy in granulomatosis with polyangiitis (Wegeners). Results of a single-center cohort study on 66 patients. J Autoimmun 2014;50:135–41.

48. Cartin-Ceba R, Golbin J, Keogh KA, et al. Rituximab for remission induction and maintenance in refractory granulomatosis with polyangiitis (Wegener's): a single-center ten-year experience. Arthritis Rheum 2012;64:3770–8.

49. Walsh M, Flossmann O, Berden A, et al. Risk factors for relapse of antineutrophil cytoplasmic antibody-associated vasculitis. Arthritis Rheum 2012;64:542–8.

50. Available at: http://www.cdc.gov/mmwr/preview/mmwrhtml/mm6104a9.htm. Accessed November 20, 2014.

51. Miyakis S, Lockshin MD, Atsumi T, et al. International consensus statement on an update of the classification criteria for definite antiphospholipid syndrome (APS). J Thromb Haemost 2006;4:295–306.

52. Erkan D, Lockshin MD. Non-criteria manifestations of antiphospholipid syndrome. Lupus 2010;19:424–7.

53. Lie JT. Vasculopathy of the antiphospholipid syndromes revisited: thrombosis is the culprit and vasculitis the consort. Lupus 1996;5:368–71.

54. Gertner E. Diffuse alveolar hemorrhage in the antiphospholipid syndrome: spectrum of disease and treatment. J Rheumatol 1999;26:805–7.

55. Asherson RA, Cervera R, Wells AU. Diffuse alveolar hemorrhage: a nonthrombotic antiphospholipid lung syndrome? Semin Arthritis Rheum 2005;35:138–42.

56. Espinosa G, Cervera R, Font J, et al. The lung in the antiphospholipid syndrome. Ann Rheum Dis 2002;61:195–8.

57. Cartin-Ceba R, Peikert T, Ashrani A, et al. Primary antiphospholipid syndrome-associated diffuse alveolar hemorrhage. Arthritis Care Res (Hoboken) 2014;66: 301–10.

58. Deane KD, West SG. Antiphospholipid antibodies as a cause of pulmonary capillaritis and diffuse alveolar hemorrhage: a case series and literature review. Semin Arthritis Rheum 2005;35:154–65.

59. Hellmark T, Segelmark M. Diagnosis and classification of Goodpasture's disease (anti-GBM). J Autoimmun 2014;49:108–12.

60. Pedchenko V, Bondar O, Fogo AB, et al. Molecular architecture of the Goodpasture autoantigen in anti-GBM nephritis. N Engl J Med 2010;363:343–54.

61. Herody M, Bobrie G, Gouarin C, et al. Anti-GBM disease: predictive value of clinical, histological and serological data. Clin Nephrol 1993;40:249–55.

62. Lazor R, Bigay-Gamé L, Cottin V, et al. Alveolar hemorrhage in anti-basement membrane antibody disease: a series of 28 cases. Medicine (Baltimore) 2007; 86:181–93.

63. Merkel F, Pullig O, Marx M, et al. Course and prognosis of anti-basement membrane antibody (anti-BM-Ab)-mediated disease: report of 35 cases. Nephrol Dial Transplant 1994;9:372–6.

64. Min SA, Rutherford P, Ward MK, et al. Goodpasture's syndrome with normal renal function. Nephrol Dial Transplant 1996;11:2302–5.

65. Levy JB, Turner AN, Rees AJ, et al. Long-term outcome of anti-glomerular basement membrane antibody disease treated with plasma exchange and immunosuppression. Ann Intern Med 2001;134:1033–42.

66. Moroni G, Ponticelli C. Rapidly progressive crescentic glomerulonephritis: early treatment is a must. Autoimmun Rev 2014;13:723–9.
67. Dammacco F, Battaglia S, Gesualdo L, et al. Goodpasture's disease: a report of ten cases and a review of the literature. Autoimmun Rev 2013;12:1101–8.
68. Pusey CD, Levy JB. Plasmapheresis in immunologic renal disease. Blood Purif 2012;33:190–8.
69. Johnson JP, Whitman W, Briggs WA, et al. Plasmapheresis and immunosuppressive agents in antibasement membrane antibody-induced Goodpasture's syndrome. Am J Med 1978;64:354–9.
70. Syeda UA, Singer NG, Magrey M. Anti-glomerular basement membrane antibody disease treated with rituximab: a case-based review. Semin Arthritis Rheum 2013;42:567–72.
71. Srivastava A, Rao GK, Segal PE, et al. Characteristics and outcome of crescentic glomerulonephritis in patients with both antineutrophil cytoplasmic antibody and anti-glomerular basement membrane antibody. Clin Rheumatol 2013; 32:1317–22.
72. Cui Z, Zhao J, Jia XY, et al. Anti-glomerular basement membrane disease: outcomes of different therapeutic regimens in a large single-center Chinese cohort study. Medicine (Baltimore) 2011;90:303–11.
73. Rutgers A, Slot M, van Paassen P, et al. Coexistence of anti-glomerular basement membrane antibodies and myeloperoxidase-ANCAs in crescentic glomerulonephritis. Am J Kidney Dis 2005;46:253–62.
74. Hamuryudan V, Er T, Seyahi E, et al. Pulmonary artery aneurysms in Behçet syndrome. Am J Med 2004;117:867–70.
75. Seyahi E, Melikoglu M, Akman C, et al. Pulmonary artery involvement and associated lung disease in Behçet disease: a series of 47 patients. Medicine (Baltimore) 2012;91:35–48.
76. Hassine E, Bousnina S, Marniche K, et al. Pulmonary artery aneurysms in Behçet's disease: contribution of imaging in 5 cases. Ann Med Interne (Paris) 2002;153:147–52.
77. Emad Y, Abdel-Razek N, Gheita T, et al. Multislice CT pulmonary findings in Behçet's disease (report of 16 cases). Clin Rheumatol 2007;26:879–84.
78. Trad S, Bensimhon L, El Hajjam M, et al. 18F-fluorodeoxyglucose-positron emission tomography scanning is a useful tool for therapy evaluation of arterial aneurysm in Behçet's disease. Joint Bone Spine 2013;80:420–3.
79. Uzun O, Akpolat T, Erkan L. Pulmonary vasculitis in Behcet disease: a cumulative analysis. Chest 2005;127:2243–53.
80. Hatemi G, Yazici Y, Yazici H. Behçet's syndrome. Rheum Dis Clin North Am 2013; 39:245–61.
81. Saadoun D, Asli B, Wechsler B, et al. Long-term outcome of arterial lesions in Behçet disease: a series of 101 patients. Medicine (Baltimore) 2012;91:18–24.
82. Schreiber BE, Noor N, Juli CF, et al. Resolution of Behçet's syndrome associated pulmonary arterial aneurysms with infliximab. Semin Arthritis Rheum 2011;41:482–7.
83. Ceyran H, Akçali Y, Kahraman C. Surgical treatment of vasculo-Behçet's disease. A review of patients with concomitant multiple aneurysms and venous lesions. Vasa 2003;32:149–53.
84. Kalko Y, Basaran M, Aydin U, et al. The surgical treatment of arterial aneurysms in Behçet disease: a report of 16 patients. J Vasc Surg 2005;42:673–7.
85. Sharma S, Kamalakar T, Rajani M, et al. The incidence and patterns of pulmonary artery involvement in Takayasu's arteritis. Clin Radiol 1990;42:177–81.

86. Manganelli P, Fietta P, Carotti M, et al. Respiratory system involvement in systemic vasculitides. Clin Exp Rheumatol 2006;24:S48–59.

87. Lie JT. Isolated pulmonary Takayasu arteritis: clinicopathologic characteristics. Mod Pathol 1996;9:469–74.

88. Toledano K, Guralnik L, Lorber A, et al. Pulmonary arteries involvement in Takayasu's arteritis: two cases and literature review. Semin Arthritis Rheum 2011;41: 461–70.

89. Vanoli M, Castellani M, Bacchiani G, et al. Non-invasive assessment of pulmonary artery involvement in Takayasu's arteritis. Clin Exp Rheumatol 1999;17:215–8.

90. Arnaud L, Haroche J, Malek Z, et al. Is (18)F-fluorodeoxyglucose positron emission tomography scanning a reliable way to assess disease activity in Takayasu arteritis? Arthritis Rheum 2009;60:1193–200.

91. Addimanda O, Spaggiari L, Pipitone N, et al. Pulmonary artery involvement in Takayasu arteritis. PET/CT versus CT angiography. Clin Exp Rheumatol 2013;31: S3–4.

92. Kerr GS, Hallahan CW, Giordano J, et al. Takayasu arteritis. Ann Intern Med 1994; 120:919–29.

93. Clifford A, Hoffman GS. Recent advances in the medical management of Takayasu arteritis: an update on use of biologic therapies. Curr Opin Rheumatol 2014;26:7–15.

94. Qin L, Hong-Liang Z, Zhi-Hong L, et al. Percutaneous transluminal angioplasty and stenting for pulmonary stenosis due to Takayasu's arteritis: clinical outcome and four-year follow-up. Clin Cardiol 2009;32:639–43.

95. Hamamoto M, Futagami D. Pulmonary artery replacement for pulmonary Takayasu's arteritis. Gen Thorac Cardiovasc Surg 2012;60:435–9.

# Index

*Note:* Page numbers of article titles are in **boldface** type.

## A

Acute lupus pneumonitis, in systemic lupus erythematosus, 268–269
Airway disease, in Sjögren syndrome, 265
    in systemic lupus erythematosus, 269–270
Airway involvement, in rheumatoid arthritis, 231
Amyloidosis, pulmonary, in Sjögren syndrome, 267
Antiglomerular basement membrane antibody disease, in differential diagnosis of
    pulmonary vasculitis, 323–324
Antineutrophil cytoplasmic antibody (ANCA)-associated vasculitides, in differential
    diagnosis of pulmonary vasculitis, 317–322
Antiphospholipid syndrome, in differential diagnosis of pulmonary vasculitis, 322–323
    in systemic lupus erythematosus, 270
Aspiration pneumonitis, as complication of inflammatory myopathy, 250–251
Autologous stem cell transplantation, for ILD in systemic sclerosis, 244–245
Azathioprine, for connective tissue disease-associated ILD, 283–284
    for ILD in systemic sclerosis, 243

## B

Behcet's syndrome, 325
Beta-catenin, in pathogenesis of ILD in systemic sclerosis, 240
Biomarkers, for ILD in inflammatory myopathies, 252–255
    nonantibody, 255
    serum, 252–254
Biopsy, surgical lung, for respiratory impairment in connective tissue disease, 217
    for ILD in inflammatory myopathy, 257
Bone health measures, in management of connective tissue disease-associated
    ILD, 289
Bosentan, for ILD in systemic sclerosis, 243–244
Bronchiectasis, in rheumatoid arthritis, 231
Bronchitis, in rheumatoid arthritis, 231
Bronchoalveolar lavage, for pulmonary manifestations in Sjögren syndrome, 265
Bronchoscopy, for ILD in inflammatory myopathy, 256
    for respiratory impairment in connective tissue disease, 217

## C

Calcineurin antagonists, for connective tissue disease-associated ILD, 284–285
Cardiopulmonary rehabilitation, for connective tissue disease-associated ILD, 286
Computed tomography (CT), high-resolution, role in imaging pulmonary
    involvement in rheumatic disease, 183–186
        in diagnostic evaluation, monitoring, and prognostication, 183–185

Rheum Dis Clin N Am 41 (2015) 333–344
http://dx.doi.org/10.1016/S0889-857X(15)00020-4
0889-857X/15/$ – see front matter © 2015 Elsevier Inc. All rights reserved.

Printed and bound by CPI Group (UK) Ltd, Croydon, CR0 4YY

03/10/2024

01040497-0018